I LIVE IN MY

Kitchen

...BUT YOU DON'T HAVE TO!

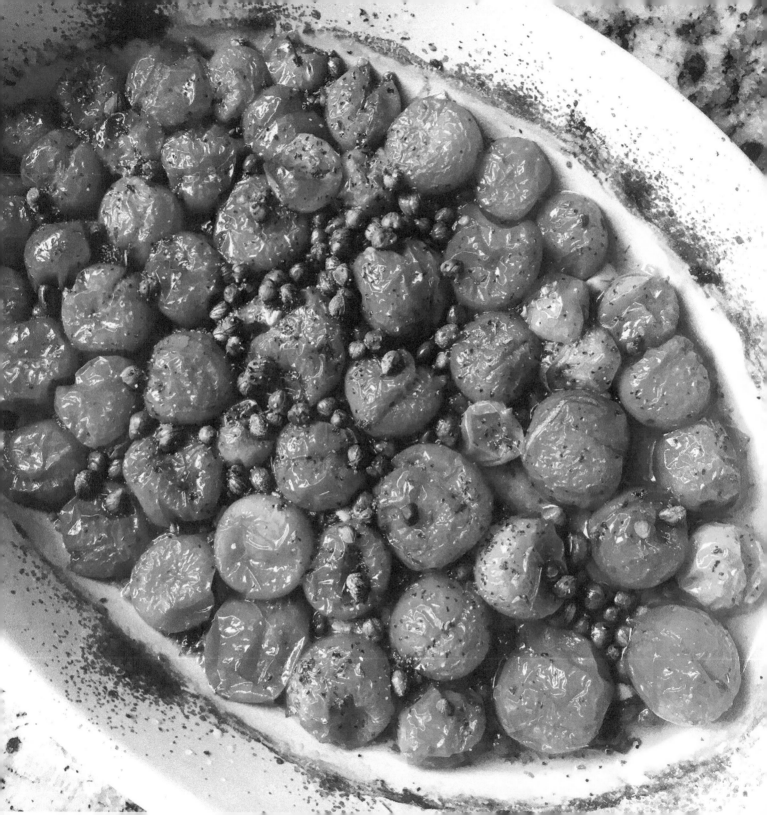

I LIVE IN MY

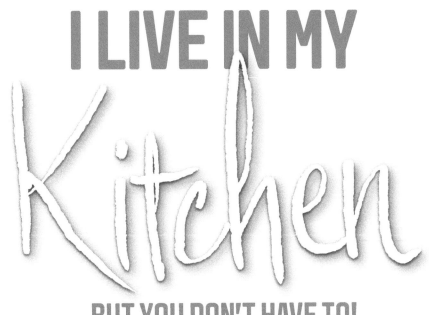

Kitchen

...BUT YOU DON'T HAVE TO!

BY ELITE JAKOB

To my Ema (mom),
who always welcomed me into her kitchen
and without judgement, let me mess up and try again -
Thank you for instilling in me
the love and appreciation for home cooking.
I love you!

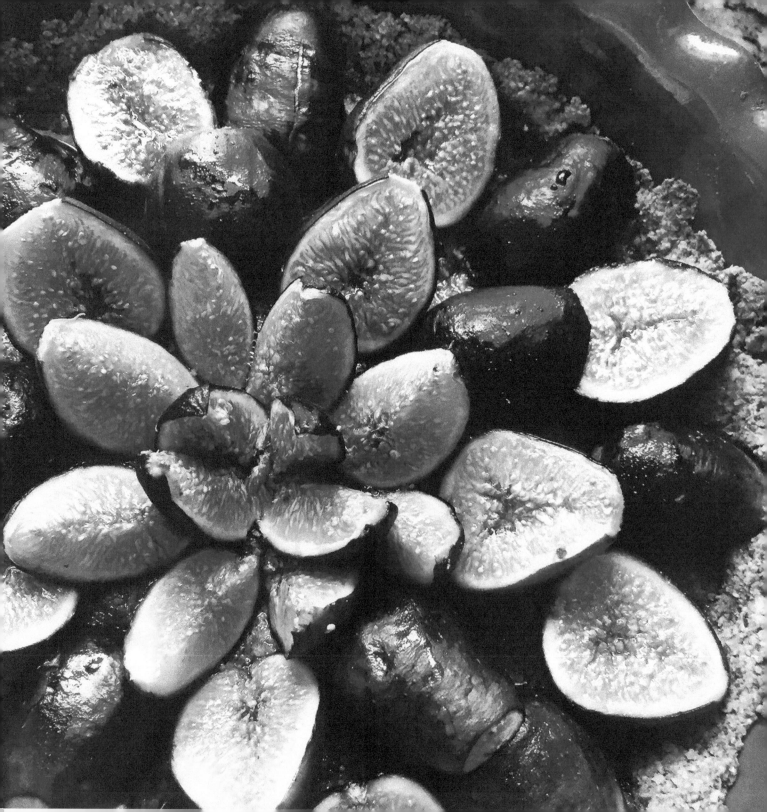

TABLE OF CONTENTS

—

I LIVE IN MY KITCHEN

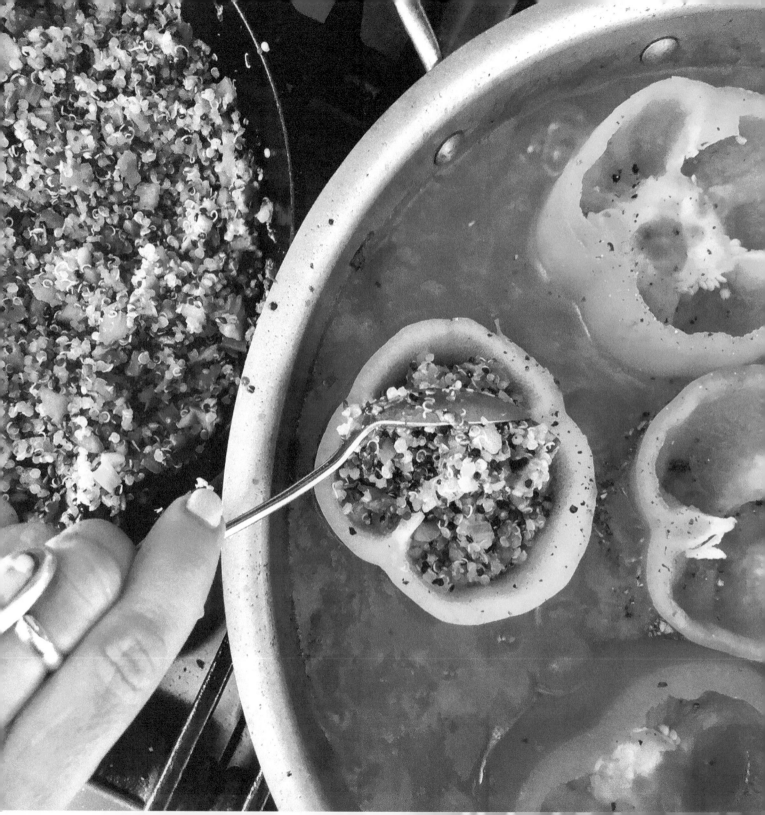

I MAY LIVE IN MY KITCHEN, BUT YOU CERTAINLY DON'T HAVE TO!

I'm on a mission to prove that anyone can cook healthy and delicious meals. With a little planning and practice—and most importantly fun—you'll learn how to cook quick and delicious meals that will fit right into your schedule.

Your nutritional gain will lead to improved energy levels, alertness, mood, digestion, and better sleep. You'll learn how to combine fresh and simple ingredients to create meals that taste delicious. Best of all, healthy food doesn't have to be boring. As your skills grow, you'll be able to create flavorful and beautiful dishes that everyone will love.

In this book, you'll find easy recipes, learn to substitute healthier ingredients without compromising the taste of the dishes, learn healthy dietary practices and tips, and learn how to stock your kitchen with cooking and baking essentials. This book will inspire you to get in the kitchen to take better care of yourself and your loved ones.

The recipes in this book are my template for healthy living. They're based on good fats, whole grains (mainly gluten-free), a lot of fruits and vegetables, selective animal products, and spices that can be easily found in any food store. There are NO recipes using white flour, refined white sugar, corn products, peanuts, soy, processed ingredients, chemicals, artificial sweeteners, preservatives, or food dyes. When your kitchen is stocked with wholesome ingredients that support your health, you'll find it easy to cook and eat healthy.

Anyone can use this book, no matter where you fall on this spectrum:
- The rookie cook who needs a few "staple" recipes that are simple and delicious
- The middle of the road cook, who is ready to "step it up" with new and delicious recipes that still take little time to prepare
- The experienced cook, who is looking for new recipes with healthier and more wholesome ingredients.

HOW I ENDED UP IN THE KITCHEN

Growing up in Israel, food was a central component of our culture and everyday lives. Typical Israeli cuisine, some 40 years ago, revolved around fruits, vegetables, eggs, dairy and breads. We ate a little meat, mainly chicken. Pre-packaged snack foods and processed foods were scarce. We used locally-sourced ingredients to prepare seasonal foods, a style similar to what we now call "farm to table."

Food didn't travel long distances, and since Israel is a small country, we generally knew exactly where our food came from. To this day, my mom gets her eggs from a friend who owns a chicken coop in a neighboring town, and fresh olive oil from another friend who lives 15 minutes away.

My mom (in Hebrew we called her, "Ema,") used to pack us a wholesome lunch – a sandwich with soft cheese and pitted olives, or half a pita bread with Hummus and cut-up pickles. She would include a side or two of whole fruits and vegetables such as clementines, tomatoes or cucumbers. Food was simpler and healthier then.

Most of the foods we ate were homemade. My Ema had cooking sessions in the kitchen once or twice a week, preparing a few dishes in large quantities that would last several days. We were always well-fed, but I sometimes resented how little we ate at restaurants. Little did I know, that this was the healthier option! My Ema cooked around her work and home life, creating meals as well as snacks, so we always had healthy options available in the refrigerator and pantry. She made pickles, pickled herring, hummus, tahini, salads, tomato sauce, jams, baked goods, and so much more. Many of the recipes in this book are inspired by my mom's cooking, and my first attempts to recreate some of her vast repertoire.

Even when I was a young girl, Ema welcomed me into her kitchen. She never complained about my interruptions, or any additional mess. Slowly but surely, I became very comfortable in the kitchen. When it was my parents' turn to host their circle of friends, my job was to bake. Ema and I would go all-out, researching recipes weeks ahead of time. It was almost a competition - the quest to develop the best menu and find unique recipes to impress our guests. We had a lot of fun.

My mother allowed me to experiment in the kitchen and expand my skills without judgment. When I made mistakes—and trust me, I made plenty—she didn't get upset. She would shrug and say, "It's just a cake, no big deal, let's make another one." The more I practiced, the more comfortable and confident I became in the kitchen. To this day, I still experiment and learn. What's the worst that can happen? Seriously!

WHY SHOULD YOU GET IN THE KITCHEN?

At this point you might be saying, "But I like eating out!" Me too. Don't get me wrong, I still go out to eat. I love to dress up, meet friends and family, and have a good time without having to do the dishes. It's a fun break. But for the health of my body, I can't eat out often. In a restaurant, I never know exactly what goes into the food and how it's cooked. Even the best restaurants may use chemicals to tenderize a chicken, or use low-grade oil to cook my food. These kinds of hidden ingredients can be harmful to our health, particularly if we consume too much of them.

One of the biggest culprits in restaurant food is table salt. In order to make food more flavorful and appealing, many restaurants add a lot of salt to their dishes. Worse still, they use table salt (the cheapest kind), which is heavily processed, bleached, and lacks the natural, healthy minerals of sea salt. When you cook at home, you can use the good kind of salt like Himalayan or Celtic Sea salt, and enjoy its vast nutritional benefits.

If you eat most of your meals outside the home, or often eat carry-out or frozen food, you will not believe how much better you can feel by spending a little time in your own kitchen and eating home cooked food. If you can transition to home-cooked meals even once or twice a week, your body and mind will thank you. Even starting with small steps like packing your own lunch can have a positive effect on your health.

Homemade food is made with love and care, specifically to nourish and nurture. Restaurant food often occurs on a different scale or timeline. As a college student, I worked at a beach town as a waitress and cook, and witnessed the vibe of a restaurant kitchen. The staff and I were often tired and grumpy, and didn't care who benefitted from our meals. We just wanted to finish up with one customer and move on to the next. This type of vibe is very common behind the scenes of many restaurants, and who wants to have their food prepared by grumpy and stressed-out cooks?

By comparison, when a group of people sits down to a home-cooked meal, they know the cook cares. Home cooked meals go far beyond physical nourishment, because they nourish our souls and fill them with love. Furthermore, home-cooked meals bring families together. When people gather around the table, they're more likely to slow down to share stories, listen, laugh, catch up, and connect. Slowing down helps us to digest our food properly, as opposed to eating in a hurry, on the run or in the car. When the opportunity arises and you can have a family dinner, grab it! Obviously, home-cooked meals can be challenging to prepare when life gets busy, but hopefully this book will give you some strategies to make it less challenging and more enjoyable.

THE BIG CHALLENGE

When I first moved to the States in 1989, I was excited to discover the ease of fast foods. My husband and I were busy students, subsisting mainly on boxed, bagged and processed foods. Later on, juggling work, household chores, cooking and raising three young kids was challenging and stressful. I resorted to processed food for quick and kid-friendly meals more often than ever. All I was thinking was, "Wow, how come no one ever prepared me for the challenge of feeding a family?" It might sound like a minor issue to some people, but feeding a family with healthy, tasty, easy to prepare foods was not simple at all. My son was a very picky eater and would only eat macaroni and cheese or chicken nuggets. My middle daughter had a sensitivity to milk, and my youngest would only eat French Fries and potato chips. Sadly, we ended up going to the place where they served Happy Meals, because everyone was happy there. Alternatively, I was cooking five different dishes at home every meal to satisfy everyone's dietary needs.

Change can be hard to implement, especially if we're accustomed to certain products, routines, traditions, and beliefs. I would recommend taking small steps, and being consistent when you're adopting a new change in diet or lifestyle.

LOW-FAT-LOW-SUGAR FAD

After my second daughter was born, I decided to prioritize exercise, joined a gym, and tried to eliminate all fat and sugar from my diet. After all, this was the hottest trend in those days and it became my lifestyle for a few years. I ate sugar-free, fat-free everything, and drank a lot of diet soda. With fewer calories and more exercise, I did lose some weight, but I ate little of sustenance and lots of processed foods; I was perpetually tired and developed headaches on a daily basis. I was consuming a lot of Aspartame, chemicals, food coloring, and artificial ingredients, none of which are essential nutrients. My body was craving whole foods, but I decided I needed stimulants. I leaned on caffeine and sugar for quick boosts of energy so I could continue to take care of everything and everyone. I was on a mood and energy roller coaster, and I began to gain weight again, and I felt frustrated.

BACK ON TRACK

While I thought I was taking care of myself, I didn't realize how my lifestyle habits caused my wellbeing to decline. I found myself reading a lot about nutrition and different dietary styles people adopt. I was mostly interested in learning about the connection between the food we eat and our health. One of the theories that caught my attention was the Paleo Diet, consisting of organic and free-range animal protein, eggs, vegetables and fruits and avoiding all processed foods, dairy, refined sugars, grains and legumes. Many people choose to live by this diet for health reasons, as it has been proven to help fight chronic illnesses such as Crohn, diabetes, and digestive disorders. While I didn't completely adopt this eating style, I became aware of what I was eating and how it affected my health, mood, sleep, and wellbeing. One main principle of this diet style became very clear to me; I needed to clean our diet from processed foods.

It was time to take action! I started to experiment in the kitchen, and tried new approaches to cooking for my family. It took a while, but everyone learned to love my new style of cooking and eating, and admitted that they felt better when we ate my dishes at home. For some of us, the elimination of dairy turned out to be the solution for constant bloating and discomfort.

The notion that "Food is Medicine" became a real experience for my family. This understanding led me to enroll in the Institute for Integrative Nutrition (IIN) and to become a health coach. "A certified Health Coach is a wellness authority and supportive mentor who motivates individuals to cultivate positive health choices." (www.integrativenutrition.com.) Over the year of training, I have learned about 100 dietary theories and the connection between lifestyle and wellbeing. As a result, I rediscovered my love of cooking, and wrote this cookbook to inspire others to get in the kitchen and cook for better health.

Change can be hard to implement, especially if we're accustomed to certain products, routines, traditions, and beliefs. I would recommend taking small steps, and being consistent when you're adopting a new change in diet or lifestyle. For my family and myself, the first step towards a healthier lifestyle was to eliminate all sweetened soft drinks and diet sodas at home. Of course, I had a lot of resistance from my kids so I introduced the changes slowly. First, I bought less of those drinks and we had them only on weekends or special dinners at home. Later, I stopped completely to bring them home and the kids only had them when we ate out. Eventually, as their taste buds changed, they began to dislike the overpoweringly chemical sweet taste and switched to drinking water. We continue to make small changes and discover new foods and healthier options that enable us to do what we enjoy. Our lifestyle now supports our lives.

ONE PERSON'S FOOD IS ANOTHER PERSON'S POISON

We're all individuals. Each of us has different dietary needs, food sensitivities, lifestyle preferences, religious beliefs, and other factors that affect our meals. Yet none of us should base our diet on highly-processed or genetically-modified foods. Nor should we consume additives, dyes, foods containing growth hormones, pesticides, or any other artificial ingredients with names so long, they can't be pronounced. As our diets include more whole foods, we'll feel better, gain resistance to chronic diseases and illnesses, and ultimately maintain a healthier weight. The recipes in this book consist of nutritious ingredients recombined into a range of foods from appetizers to desserts, including vegetarian and animal-based dishes. It's my hope that these recipes inspire you to continue to make small changes to better your health.

EATING HEALTHY IS A LIFESTYLE, NOT A DIET

When someone says he or she is on a 'diet', it usually means that they are on a temporary program that lasts a few weeks, rather than a sustainable way of life. Instead of a diet, we can adopt a healthy lifestyle that will be easy to sustain for life. Some people find that eating healthy all week and 'cheating' a little on a weekend is doable for them. Or, having a small treat once a day is another way to manage and not feel deprived. It's not what you do once in a while that determines your health, but what you do most of the time.

The rule of 80/20 is another way to make a healthy lifestyle easier to sustain. This rule allows us to consume wholesome and healthy foods—fruits and vegetables, organic animal products and healthy grains—most of the time (80%). The 20% allows for infrequent "cheating" with foods you crave, like desserts, baked goods, and other processed foods. After all, it's very challenging to eat clean and healthy all the time, so be gentle on yourself and allow for some cheating with foods you crave.

Pursuing health and a sustainable lifestyle is a way of life. You can eat healthy even when you're traveling for work or vacation. Many restaurants nowadays will accommodate customers' requests, such as serving dressing on the side or substituting side dishes with vegetables or a salad. Clean food is more accessible than ever before for the consumer. Most food stores today allocate shelf space for healthy foods and a special section for organic produce.

PLAN, PREPARE, AND LOSE STRESS

When my kids were young, they used to ask me on the way home from school "What's for dinner?" I hated that question. I remember it used to cause a moment of panic for me, especially if I had no clue what we are going to have for dinner that night. But when I did have a plan, it was much easier to handle. For many of us, it's not feasible to go to the grocery store every day, or start planning dinner 20 minutes before everyone gets hungry. We've all been there and know that it simply doesn't work. To avoid this stressful situation, I've come up with my own tricks to survive the 'What's for dinner' panic mode.

My list of staples will help you stay prepared, so you'll be able to cook even when your life gets crazy busy. First of all, you'll need to recognize that food preparation is a priority in your life. Advance preparation saves cooking time, and saving time often means less stress. You can benefit from planning meals a day ahead, which may mean pulling something out of the freezer in the morning or chopping part of the recipe ahead of time. Yes, you may need to manage your time a bit differently or increase your scheduling and organizational skills, but the benefits can reach beyond the kitchen. Sometimes, I place a couple of ingredients on my counter at night, to "get me going" in the right direction the following day. Once you have the ingredients on hand, you can relax, because all of the recipes in this book are super-easy to prepare.

Another strategy to keep stress out of the kitchen for me was to create a "favorite meals" list and hang it on a board for everyone to see. Everyone can be involved in creating a list of about 10-14 favorite dishes, and you can make this into a rotating menu with a variety of ingredients. This allows you to plan weeks in advance, my kids loved to look at the list and know "what's for dinner," and I loved having a plan and no stress.

KEEP IT CLEAN AND SIMPLE

You don't have to be a trained chef in order to cook delicious meals that will nourish your body and soul. The recipes in this book are based on easy-to-find ingredients and straightforward steps. There's no need to crowd your kitchen with appliances and gadgets, either. Please see the "Tools" section for my recommendations; you can keep your working kitchen simple and clear, just like the recipes in this book. My recipes follow the concept of clean eating, which simply means eating whole foods, or 'real' foods, that are minimally processed and refined, using natural spices to create an assortment of flavors.

BUY SIMPLY, TOO

Grocery shopping is a crucial first step to healthy living. With the abundance of packaged foods, frozen meals, targeted marketing, and a busy life, it's no wonder we end up filling our homes with too much processed foods instead of wholesome and healthy options. The food industry uses very smart marketing techniques to make us believe we are buying a healthy product and therefore making our decision very complicated. That is why reading labels is essential when trying to eat real and clean foods. When purchasing groceries, look at the ingredient list on the back package. Ideally, the list should be five items or less and consists of items you recognize rather than hard to pronounce chemicals. After all, what ends up in your shopping cart will end up in your kitchen, and inevitably in your or your family's body. Fill up your refrigerator, pantry, and everyone's lunch boxes with fresh, wholesome, and healthy food choices and you will be on your way to healthy living.

Take a look at the "staples" list, or even snap a photo with your phone, so you can have it on hand while you go grocery shopping. Start your shopping in the produce section. Fill your cart with fruits and vegetables in different colors and textures. Next, get a few high-quality protein options, like fish and chicken, and then move on to the frozen foods, where you may find a few fruits and vegetables in packages containing no additional ingredients. It's always helpful to have organic canned sources of hard-to-keep-fresh ingredients, such as hearts of palm, olives, and tomatoes.

Grocery shopping is a crucial first step to healthy living. …After all, what ends up in your shopping cart will end up in your kitchen, and inevitably in your or your family's body. Fill up your refrigerator, pantry, and everyone's lunch boxes with fresh, wholesome, and healthy food choices and you will be on your way to healthy living.

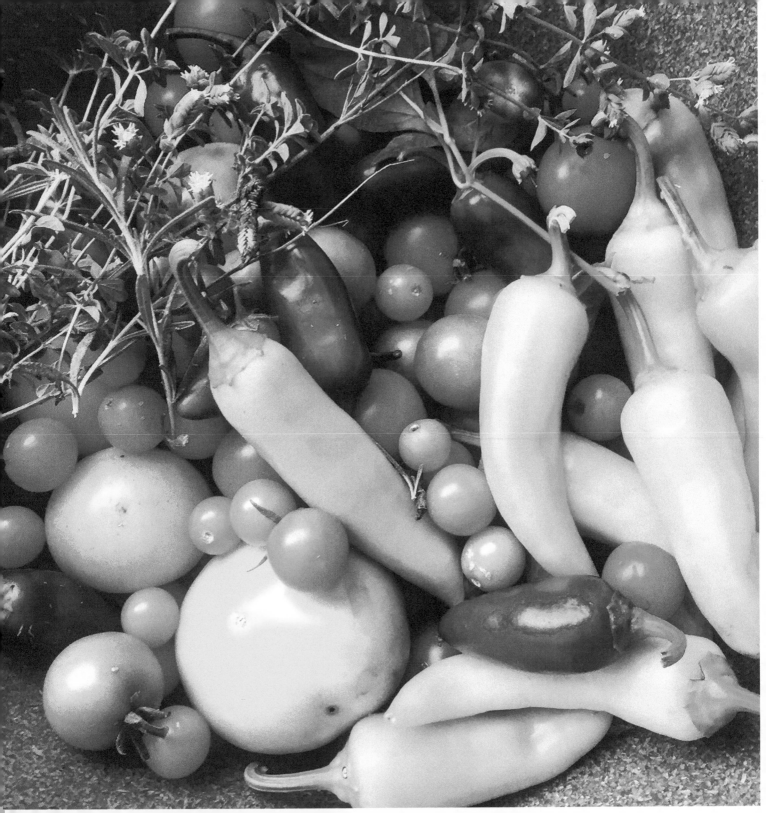

SHOPPING FOR STAPLES

Stock the best-quality items you can afford—most likely, you will use one item in multiple dishes. Shop for Certified Organic products when you can to avoid GMO (Genetically Modified Organisms), pesticides, hormones, antibiotics, synthetic chemicals, harmful food dyes, artificially produced enhancers, artificial flavoring, and other products of modern food science. The USDA Certified Organic seal indicates that food has been grown under specific Federal guidelines. Unfortunately, the Certified Organic seal doesn't mean a product is good for your health. Certified Organic cookies and candies, for example, are still high in sugar, which could undermine your health goals. After all, organic sugar and conventional sugar are equally harmful and need to be consumed in moderation. Be a smart consumer and read labels.

Food cost is always a consideration, whether you're feeding yourself or a group. Organic and high quality products tend to be more expensive than conventional items, which can complicate your choices. However, when you buy fewer pre-packaged foods and more 'clean' foods, you'll save money. My list does not include juices, soda, pre packaged snack bags, cereal boxes, bottled salad dressings, and many other items that add to the grocery bill. Moreover, today's companies are manufacturing more wholesome products to meet consumer demand, which is slowly leading to lower prices. When you find products that work for you and your family, you may be able to buy them in bulk, to lower the unit cost. In the long run, buying high-quality ingredients will turn out to be a good investment. If you allow "fast" or convenience foods to dominate your diet and your pantry, the end cost to your health can be astronomical.

My list of staples will help you stay prepared, so you'll be able to cook even when your life gets crazy busy. ... Once you have the ingredients on hand, you can relax, because all of the recipes in this book are super-easy to prepare.

PRODUCE

To begin your shopping journey, here are two helpful lists published by the EWG (Environmental Working Group, www.ewg.org) The "Dirty Dozen," a list of fruits and vegetables that—when grown conventionally—contain high levels of pesticides and toxins. The second list, the "Clean Fifteen," lists fifteen fruits and vegetables that are safe to buy conventionally, since they contain few or no pesticides and toxins. EWG's 2016 Shopper's Guide to Pesticides in Produce™

The Dirty Dozen:	Tomatoes	Clean Fifteen:	Papayas
(buy organic to	Sweet bell peppers	*(Safe to buy*	Kiwi
avoid pesticides)	Cherry tomatoes	*non-organic)*	Eggplant
Strawberries	Cucumbers	Avocadoes	Honeydew melon
Apples	Snap peas	Sweet corn	Grapefruits
Nectarines	Blueberries	Pineapples	Cantaloupe
Peaches	Potatoes	Cabbage	Cauliflower
Celery	Hot peppers	Sweet peas (frozen)	
Grapes	Lettuce	Onions	
Cherries	Kale/collard greens	Asparagus	
Spinach	Green beans	Mangos	

DAIRY

Dairy can be problematic food for many people. Milk protein, known as casein, can be difficult to digest and may cause adverse reactions including skin rashes, eczema, asthma, allergies, bloating, and digestive upset. While advertising claims "milk is good for you," conventional or commercially-available milk contains antibiotics and hormones that can cause even greater health issues. If you decide to include dairy in your diet, look for certified organic, full-fat products. Full-fat dairy is less processed than the low or no-fat varieties. I've also included grass-fed butter and organic kefir in this shopping list, as both foods contain very little dairy protein but are rich in nutrients.

RECOMMENDED STAPLES LIST

The list below can help you organize your kitchen and stock it with healthy ingredients to prepare recipes in this book and beyond. You don't have to have all of the ingredients in each category, a few will do, but you can refer to this list as the healthy choice in each category.

OILS

Coconut oil

Extra Virgin Olive oil
(not for cooking)

Ghee (clarified butter)

Grass fed butter

Olive oil (for light cooking)

SPICES

Make sure they are pure, with no additives

Cumin, curry, garlic powder, onion powder, oregano, paprika, pepper, rosemary, sea salt, thyme, turmeric, cayenne pepper, chili pepper.

MEAT / POULTRY / EGGS

Have on hand or in the freezer two packages of organic:

Bone-in chicken breasts, drumsticks, or quarters.

Chicken tenders

Skinless, boneless chicken breasts or thighs

Whole chicken

Grass-fed beef, or ground or pieces

Free-range organic eggs (pastured if available)

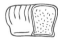

BREAD

Any organic bread

Homemade bread

FISH

Wild Caught is recommended

Cod

Halibut

Salmon

Swordfish

Tuna

CONDIMENTS

Almond butter

Cashew butter

Apple cider vinegar

Coconut amino or organic soy sauce

Hummus

Mustard

Capers

Kosher pickles

Olives

Roasted peppers (in a jar)

Salsa

Sun-dried tomatoes

Sunflower seed butter

Vegetable broth (organic)

NUTS

Choose raw nuts and seeds to avoid added oils, sugars, or salt

Almonds, Brazil nuts, cashews, macadamia nuts, pecans, pine nuts, pistachios, walnuts

SEEDS

Chia seeds, flax seeds, hemp seeds (raw, shelled), pumpkin seeds, quinoa, sesame seeds, sunflower seeds

PRODUCE

Have on hand a few fruits & vegetables at all times:

Apples
Asparagus
Avocados
Bananas
Beets
Berries
Bok choy
Brussels sprouts
Cabbage
Carrots
Cauliflower
Celery
Colorful mix of bell peppers
Cucumbers
Garlic
Herbs

Leafy greens like baby spinach, kale, mixed greens, mixed lettuce, etc.
Lemons
Tomatoes/Mini tomatoes
Onions
Radishes
Sweet potatoes

DAIRY

Organic is preferred

Full-fat goat cheese
Full-fat feta cheese
Full-fat mozzarella cheese
Grass-fed butter
Kefir

GRAINS

Look for high quality and organic grains

Rice
Buckwheat
Millet
Oats
Sprouted rice

FLOUR AND SUGAR

Look for high quality and organic grains

Almond flour
Arrowroot flour
Coconut flour
Flaxseed meal
Spelt flour
Einkorn flour
Emmer flour
Raw honey
Raw maple syrup
Coconut sugar
Stevia (organic)

CANNED FOOD

Look for BPA-free, organic cans

Artichoke hearts
Chickpeas
Coconut milk
Hearts of palm
Pizza sauce
Salmon (wild-caught)
Sardines in olive oil or water
Stewed tomatoes
Tomato sauce

FROZEN FOODS

Organic frozen produce is available in many food stores

Berries, broccoli florets, cauliflower, eggplant, figs, green beans, kale, mango, okra, organic rice, pineapple, spinach, zucchini

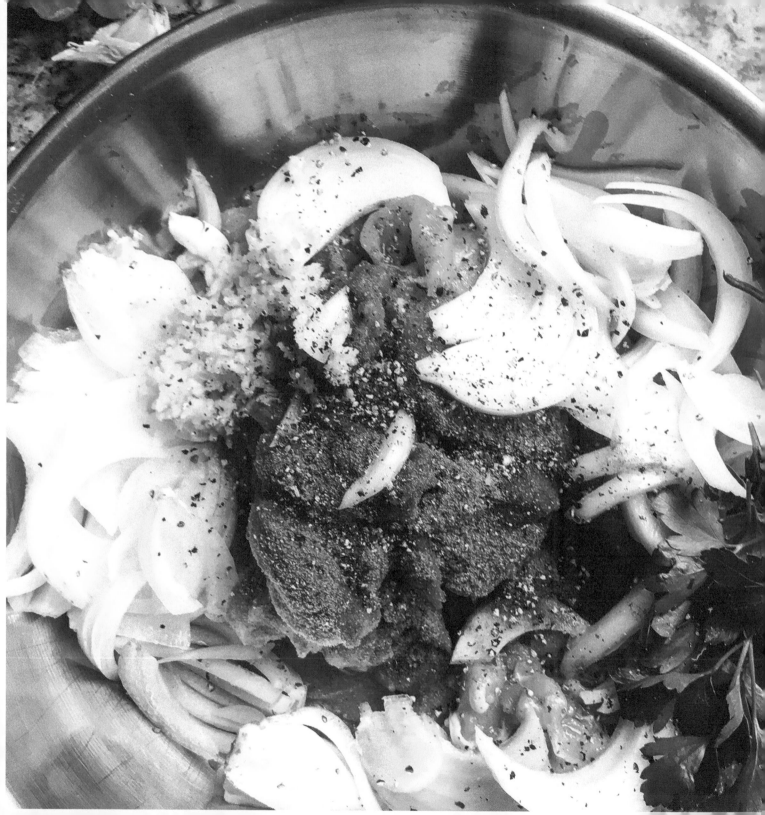

COOKING METHODS AND TIPS

Many of my dishes are made using a similar technique. I start off with a large skillet on the stove (most commonly with coconut oil), and continue adding ingredients slowly to create the dish. When I create a recipe, I'm trying to avoid as many dishes and steps as possible so the recipes stay simple and quick. As you scroll throughout the book, you'll find this technique repeating itself because it works! Even when I use the food processor, I try to 'layer' the ingredients in a way that will save time and clean up.

When it comes to cooking, I often encourage people to "make it their own" or "wing it." What do I mean by that? I believe in following a recipe that you like, but at the same time not feeling like you have to follow it strictly to a T. Cooking recipes are OK to play with!

However, for baking I'd recommend following the recipe exactly. Baking is more like a chemical interaction of the ingredients, while cooking can be flexible and fun.

Cooking is simple, and I encourage you to substitute ingredients whenever you feel it's appropriate, either because you don't have an ingredient on hand or maybe because you and your family dislike an item in the recipe. For example, instead of parsley you can use cilantro or vice versa. Instead of cumin, use garlic powder or curry, or don't add anything at all. I promise you that the dish won't be much different if you make minor changes. You know best what your family likes and dislikes, so use spices accordingly. At the same time, don't be afraid of introducing new flavors, one spice or new vegetable at a time. I find that exposing children to a variety of flavors from a young age helps them become more comfortable with different types of food. This cookbook gives you the knowledge and skills to keep food healthy, so use these tools to make sure any substitution is a healthy one.

HAVE FUN WITH IT!

The main focus of this book is for you to learn how to love cooking and have fun in the kitchen. Leave the stress outside the kitchen, because cooking should never become a source of stress! Start with baby steps and choose easy recipes because usually the tastiest dishes are the simple ones. The more you practice, the more comfortable you'll be, and the more fun you'll have in the kitchen. Cooking is a learning process just like any other skill we acquire. I too, learn something about cooking everyday, whether on the Internet, television, travel, or simply talking with friends about food. It's also a creative act where you can express yourself and your taste with the food you prepare. Dare to try new things and experiment with new ingredients. Basically, if you don't burn the food, you'll end up with a great meal. The main secret is to have the right ingredients on-hand, and the rest is easy. Think of it more like "putting it together" rather than cooking.

COOK ONCE EAT TWICE

In order to maximize the time you spend in the kitchen, cook more than what you need for one meal. Either make a larger quantity of food, or several dishes at the same time. Many of my recipes are great the day of cooking, but also the day or two after. Some people call them leftovers, but I call them blessings! If you have some leftovers from dinner, they can always become lunch for the next day. You can pile a mountain of greens on a plate and top it with last night's dinner for lunch. But beware, someone in the office might eye your lunch and make it their own!

I love to have roasted chicken as leftovers so I can make a delicious homemade chicken salad the day or two after. Some leftovers can be jazzed up a bit and become the next day's dinner. For example, vegetable dishes can be warmed up and put on rice or quinoa and become a satisfying, delicious meal tomorrow. Roasted vegetables are great to make a frittata the day after. Or, chop chicken or fish, add chopped vegetables on the side and create your own taco dinner using large green leaves or taco shells as wraps. Food in the fridge keeps fresh for a couple of days, so don't feel like you're giving your family and loved ones 'bad' food. In fact, some dishes, such as stews and brisket, even taste better the next day or two after cooking, as the meat becomes even more tender and soaked with flavors.

COOKWARE TO USE

I like to keep my cookware simple, as well. My two main go-to cookware items are cast iron skillets, and high-quality stainless steel ones. In this book, you'll come across many recipes, from savory dishes to sweet ones, using these two.

I often use my high-quality 12" skillet (with a lid) because of how versatile it is in my kitchen. It is large enough to fit a one-dish meal, easy to clean, can be transferred from the stove to the oven, safe for our health, perfect for storing food overnight and warm up the next day. It makes life easier in the kitchen and well worth the (small) investment

Next are my cast-iron skillets. I love them so much that I had to get three of them, in case three dishes are going on at the same time, which is the case most of the time in our kitchen. As we now know, coated pans are not safe for us, because of the possibility of them releasing toxins into our foods. Start with one skillet at a time and get a feel for how to use them. I personally think that food tastes better when prepared in cast-iron skillets. We use them for roasting vegetables, searing meat and chicken, frying eggs, and even baking cakes as they're very versatile. Lastly, they're affordable, which makes the transition much easier for everyone.

Cooking with cast iron takes a bit of a practice and adjustment, but once you get used to it, it's a breeze. You can't put cast iron in the dishwasher, or use dish soap on them. Once they're washed, you must dry them with a towel and spread some kind of cooking oil thinly on the surface to prevent rusting. This is called seasoning the pan. The more you use cast iron cookware, the better they become, and the easier cleanup gets.

Other useful cookware to have in the kitchen:
- 9x13" Oven-safe ceramic or glass dish
- 12" Oven-safe round ceramic or glass dish
- Muffins tin (minis and regular size)
- Rolling pin
- 2 Cutting boards (glass or bamboo are preferred)
- Strainer
- 4-5 Spatulas
- Potato masher
- Chicken shears
- 1 Set of good knives
- Soup pot
- Sauce pot
- 2 Cookie sheets
- Mixer
- Blender
- Hand held blender
- 2-3 Skillets

THE FAT TRUTH

For the longest time, Fat has been viewed as the enemy in our diet causing weight gain and diseases. However, recent research and studies have shown that not all fats are created equally, and certain fats are important to include in our diet for optimal health. With so much conflicting information out there about fat, no wonder we are so confused about this issue. Let's explore briefly what fats are good for us and which ones are bad and best to avoid.

Bad fats include: all processed oils like safflower, soybean, sunflower, corn and cottonseed; hydrogenated and partially hydrogenated oil; margarine and shortening. Bad animal fats include fat that comes from feedlot animal meat; non-organic poultry; and fat from conventional dairy products.

Good fats include: coconut oil and butter; olive oil; flaxseed oil; avocado oil. Good animal fats include grass fed and organic lamb and beef; organic chicken, duck and turkey; pasture-raised eggs; wild caught fish, sardines, herring, trout and salmon. Grass fed butter, ghee; nuts and seed; nut butter; avocados and olives.*

In broad terms, we want to avoid the bad fats because they contain high levels of omega-6, pesticides and hormones, and they can cause inflammation, and increase the risk of heart disease. On the other hand, good fats are an important part of our diet because they provide us with essential building blocks and can increase metabolism, stimulate fat burning, cut hunger, optimize cholesterol profile, potentially reverse diabetes and reduce the risk for heat disease.

*Dr. Mark Hyman www.drhyman.com

WHICH OIL TO USE AND WHEN

We were told for years that vegetable oil is good for us, but the truth is that these light yellow clear oils are highly processed and contain high levels of Omega-6, which are highly inflammatory and harmful to our health. Switching to healthier oil options is a fairly easy switch that I recommend implementing right away for better health.**

OILS AND FATS

Coconut Oil: Use coconut oil for any cooking job, baking, and sautéing. Coconut oil is packed with nutrients and anti-inflammatory properties and it doesn't burn easily. It's a good practice to keep a jar by the stove for easy access and everyday cooking and baking needs.

Refined vs. Unrefined Coconut Oil: Refined coconut oil doesn't have a pronounced coconut flavor, whereas unrefined does. They're both healthy choices for cooking and baking, so it's really a matter of personal taste. Both kinds will keep well in room temperature and you can scoop them right out of the jar.

Olive Oil: Besides being very healthy, olive oil adds a lot of flavor to our food. Use extra virgin olive oil in any dish that doesn't require high temperature cooking, like salads and other cold dishes. Use regular olive oil and coconut oil for higher temperature cooking, but coconut oil is preferred for higher temperatures cooking. Make sure your olive oil is packed in a dark container to preserve its quality, marked "certified organic," and fresh.

Grass-Fed Butter: Forget everything you've heard about butter in the past, it's actually a good source of fat for our body and brain. Make sure the butter you buy is organic and from grass-fed sources. Use it for spreading, baking and light cooking. Butter can replace all margarines and other "taste like butter" spreads.

Ghee: Ghee is the fat portion of the butter, containing almost no dairy components. It is great in cooking and considered to be good fat. It contains essential nutrients and has rich flavors.

**Dr. Mark Hyman: *Why Vegetable Oils Should Not Be Part of Your Diet*

Sugars and Other Sweeteners

Coconut Sugar: Use coconut sugar instead of regular white sugar. Coconut sugar is minimally processed and contains nutrients like zinc and iron. However, it's still sugar and needs to be used in moderation.

Organic Maple Syrup: Use organic maple syrup as another alternative for white sugar, as it is minimally processed and contains nutrients like magnesium and zinc.

Raw Honey: This is another healthier alternative to white sugar. It can be used in dressings and baking, or as a sweetener for tea and oatmeal. Buy local honey if possible.

Organic Stevia: The only zero calorie sweetener that's safe for your health is organic Stevia.

Soy Sauce and Vinegar

Soy: It is currently a very controversial food among health experts. I would highly recommend reducing the use of soy and soy products to a minimum. Coconut Aminos are a good substitute for soy sauce, although it is not as salty. If you prefer to use soy sauce, organic is best.

Vinegars: Most vinegars are ok to use for cooking and dressing up a dish. Apple cider vinegar is the least processed form of vinegar, but all other types are good, in moderation. Make sure you read the label to avoid any vinegar with added chemicals.

Salt

Some of the best salts to use are Sea Salt and Himalayan Salt; they contain essential minerals and nutrients that support heart and nerve health and they are very tasty. In fact, use these kinds of salts freely on your foods, as you are benefiting from all the nutrients they supply. On the other hand, you should avoid the use of table salt at all costs! Table salt goes through a heating process, which strips it of its natural trace minerals. Many table salts even contain other chemicals that help preserve them, like bleach and dextrose (sugar).

EAT THE RAINBOW

What does it mean to eat the rainbow? It simply means eating an assortment of colored fruits and vegetables vibrant as the rainbow. Each color supplies us with unique phytochemicals, substances found only in plant foods, and potentially enhance our health. The unique phytochemicals work together with the plant's vitamins, minerals, and fiber to fight off and prevent diseases.

Plant based foods are the most important cornerstone of our health. According to the Produce for Better Health Foundation (PBH), phytochemicals may act as antioxidants, protect and regenerate essential nutrients, and/or work to deactivate cancer-causing substances. And while research has not yet determined exactly how these substances work together or which combination offers specific benefits, including a rainbow of colored plant-based foods in a diet ensures a variety of those nutrients and phytochemicals.

Since plant based food is loaded with nutrients, our goal is to consume about 75% of our daily intake from plant-based food, and the remaining 25% from animal sourced food and other sources. In general, our plate should be at least ¾ filled with plant based foods and the rest with animal based protein. When preparing a salad, try to include lots of colors along with your greens. Be creative and add different vegetables and fruits to make it healthy and fun. Add a small portion of animal-based protein such as fish, chicken or eggs, include some health fat as avocado or nuts for a complete meal. When serving colorful and beautiful dishes, you and your family will be more inclined to try them and crave for more.

 The selection and quality of foods that enters our homes starts at the grocery store or farmer's market. Look at your cart to make sure it contains a variety of colored fruits and vegetables. Start with greens and add a few other colors to create the rainbow. Be adventurous every time you're at the produce stand, and buy a vegetable or fruit you've never tried before.

It's good practice to keep rotating the types of foods you bring home and consume. This is not just to benefit from the variety of nutrients each food group has to offer, but also to ensure that your body doesn't develop an allergic reaction or other adverse reaction to one particular food you eat too much of. Even consuming too much raw kale can cause adverse reactions such as bloating or a negative effect on the thyroid. Food can be prepared in many ways; from boiling, sautéing, grilling, roasting, or simply eating food raw, each method delivers an assortment of nutritional benefits. Keep rotating between the many methods of preparing your food so you enjoy the rainbow of textures as well as nutritional values.

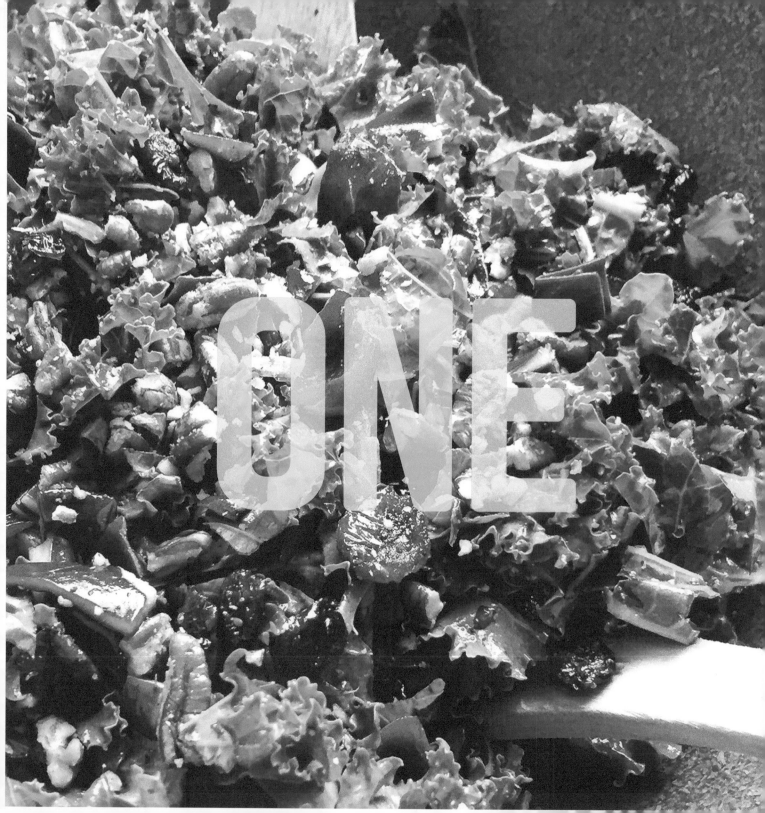

SALADS

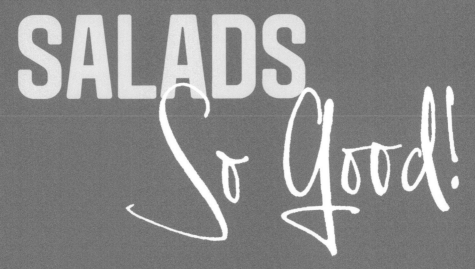

So Good!

No longer just a side dish, salads have become the main event on the dinner table. Even in restaurants, you can find salads as a main dish. Salads are a festival of flavors and colors, not just boring lettuce and tomatoes. They can be beautiful, crunchy, satisfying, and nutritious as a three-course meal. Salads are so easy to make at home and great to pack for lunch the day after. In this section, I included my go-to salads everyone will love. Most of which include one-step preparation and that is tossing everything together. Best of all, there is no stress involved when preparing a salad. All recipes include suggested quantities, but you can substitute, increase or delete an ingredient or two; make it your own and have fun with it! Whatever you do, don't forget to eat your vegetables!

ELITE'S CRUNCHY COLESLAW

This salad is a big hit in my house and a staple at any of our special meals. It is crunchy and a bit sweet and also pairs well as a side dish with everything. The original recipe calles for fried instant noodles, white sugar, canola oil, and soy sauce, none of which are used in my kitchen anymore. Here is the better-for-you version that will deliver the same flavors and crunch.

HERE IS WHAT YOU NEED:

1 bag shredded coleslaw (either plain cabbage or mixed with carrots)

1 carrot, shredded (if you are using plain shredded cabbage)

4-5 scallions, chopped

⅓ cup slivered roasted almonds

⅓ cup sunflower seeds

Dressing:

⅓ cup olive oil

⅓ cup coconut sugar

¼ cup red wine vinegar

4 tablespoons coconut aminos (or organic soy sauce)

LET'S DO THIS:

1. Combine the first 5 ingredients in a large bowl.

2. Mix the dressing very well. When ready to serve, pour over the cabbage mixture and toss well with two large spoons.

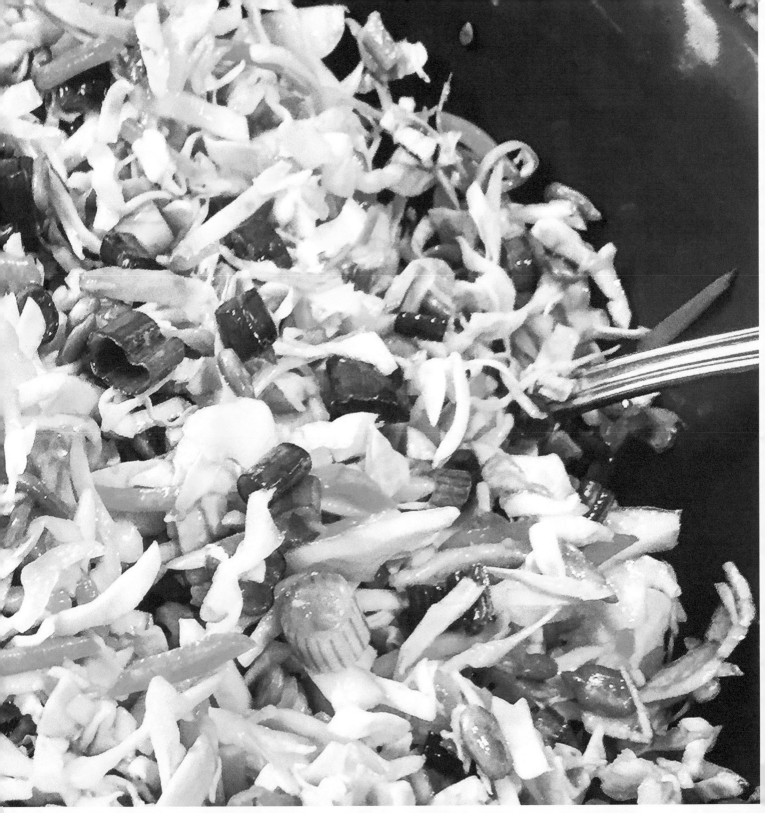

RAINBOW COLLARD GREENS & BUTTERNUT SQUASH SALAD

This is a colorful and delicious salad with a lot of flavor. The roasted butternut squash adds finesse to the bland taste of the greens and together they create a wholesome salad. Feel free to substitute the collard greens with baby spinach leaves or chopped kale.

HERE IS WHAT YOU NEED:

1 bunch rainbow collard greens, chopped

2 tablespoons oil

1 red onion, chopped

1 bag or box of greens like baby spinach, baby kale, or arugula

2 cups butternut squash, cut into small chunks

1 tablespoon olive oil

Dressing:

½ cup raw tahini

½ cup water

1 lemon, juice only

2 garlic cloves, minced

Salt and pepper

LET'S DO THIS:

1. Toss the butternut squash with 2 tablespoons of oil, sprinkle with salt and pepper, and roast it on a cookie sheet on 425°F for 25 minutes. Let cool.

2. In the meantime, layer the fresh greens on a large platter.

3. Sauté the chopped collard greens in a large skillet with olive oil. Toss a few times. Let cool. Spread on top of the fresh greens.

4. Spread the roasted butternut squash on top of all the greens.

5. Mix the dressing well and drizzle it all over the vegetables.

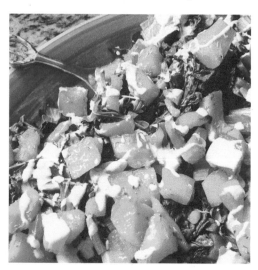

QUICK KALE & TAHINI SALAD

This salad will convert any non-kale eaters into kale addicts. It is super-easy to prepare and you can enjoy it for a couple of days. Unlike other greens, kale leaves are tough and will taste better if they sit in the dressing longer than a regular salad. Use wooden spoons or do what I do, use your hands.

HERE IS WHAT YOU NEED:

1 bunch kale, cut into
   bite-sized pieces

Dressing:

¼ cup raw tahini

¼ cup water

1" ginger, grated

2 garlic cloves, minced

1 lemon, juice only

Salt and pepper

LET'S DO THIS:

1. Place the kale in a large bowl.

2. Mix the dressing in a small bowl and pour over the kale. Work the dressing into the kale by mixing it all together for a few minutes with two wooden spoons or your hands.

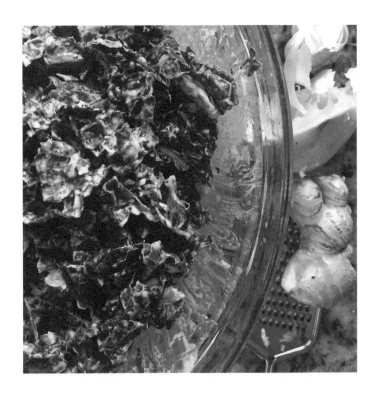

REFRESHING CARROT SALAD

Carrots are always in season, and organic carrots are so easy to find. I always have a bag in the fridge "just in case," because you can add them to nearly any dish, from a soup to a stir-fry, and even in desserts. This salad is easy to make and its vibrant color is a nice addition to any meal. It can be served as a mid-week side dish, on top of a pile of greens for lunch, or just a healthy snack option.

HERE IS WHAT YOU NEED:

1 lb. carrots, peeled and chopped into large chunks

1 onion, quartered

3 tablespoons olive oil

1 lemon, juice only

Salt and pepper

Optional: Parsley, chopped, for a garnish

LET'S DO THIS:

1. Using a food processor, process the onion and carrots until you have the consistency of rice.

2. Transfer to a bowl and season with salt, pepper, olive oil and lemon juice. Toss and serve.

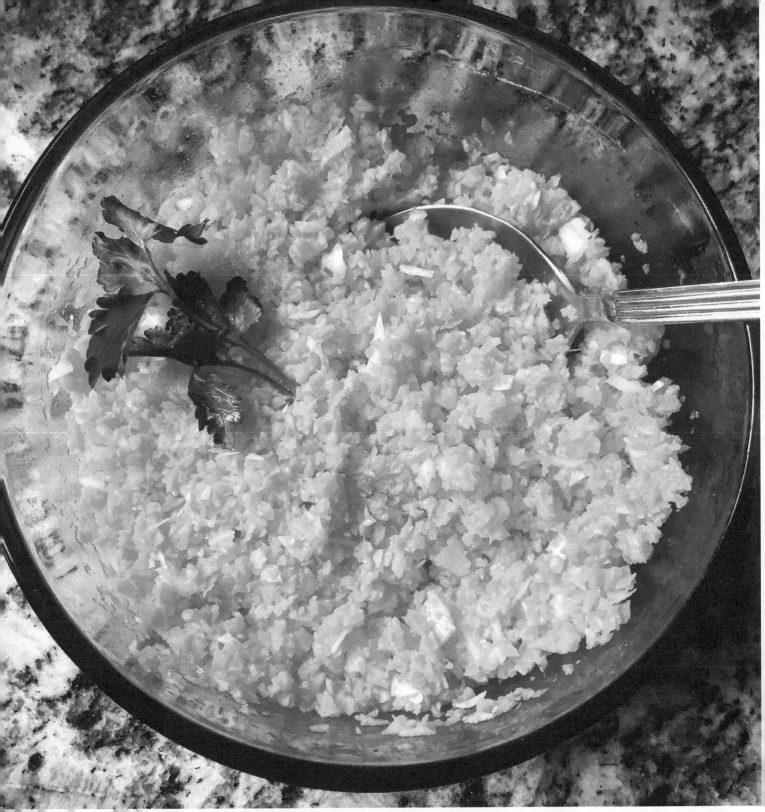

CAULIFLOWER & ARUGULA SALAD

Arugula is such a flavorful green that I always keep it on hand, either to mix with other leaves or to use it on its own. With its zingy taste and detoxifying powers, arugula is worth getting to know. This salad will keep nicely in the fridge and will make an eye candy lunch!

HERE IS WHAT YOU NEED:

1 bag shredded (2 cups) cauliflower

1 tablespoon olive oil

1 bag (or three handfuls) arugula

1 cup sun-dried or fresh cherry tomatoes, chopped

3 tablespoons olive oil

1 lemon, juice only

Salt and pepper

Optional: One handful of sunflower or pumpkin seeds, for extra crunch

LET'S DO THIS:

1. Sauté the shredded cauliflower for 4-5 minutes. Sprinkle with salt. Transfer to a large salad bowl.

2. Add the rest of the ingredients and toss well. Done!

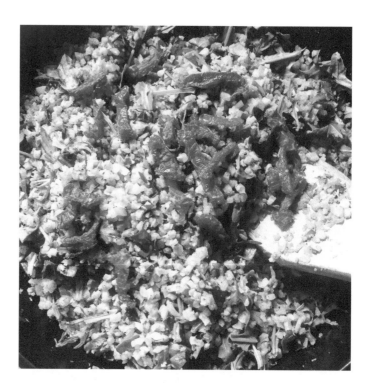

CONFETTI KALE SALAD

The beautiful colors of this salad make it the perfect dish for a potluck, or any family meal at home. The unexpected pairing of kale and apples makes for a winning combination. I promise, even the skeptics at the table will want seconds!

HERE IS WHAT YOU NEED:

1 tablespoon coconut oil

1 red onion, slivered

2 carrots, slivered

1 bunch kale, chopped into bite-size pieces

1 cup sliced apples

1 cup cooked red quinoa (½ cup dry cooked in 1 cup water)

Salt and pepper

Dressing:

1 lemon, juice only

1 tablespoon apple cider vinegar

2 tablespoons olive oil

1 tablespoon maple syrup

LET'S DO THIS:

1. In a large skillet, heat the oil and toss in the red onion, carrots and apples for a couple of minutes.

2. Add the kale and toss gently for a few seconds.

3. Transfer the mixture to a large salad bowl, add the quinoa and toss well with the dressing. Can be served right away, in room temperature or cold out of the refrigerator.

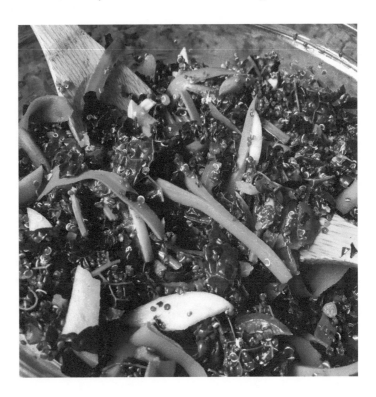

Seeds for Thought... *Quinoa is a seed (not a grain) and considered to be a Superfood. It is Gluten-free and contains iron, B-vitamins, magnesium, phosphorus, potassium, calcium, vitamin E, and fiber. It is one of a few plant foods that are considered a complete protein, containing all nine essential amino acids.*

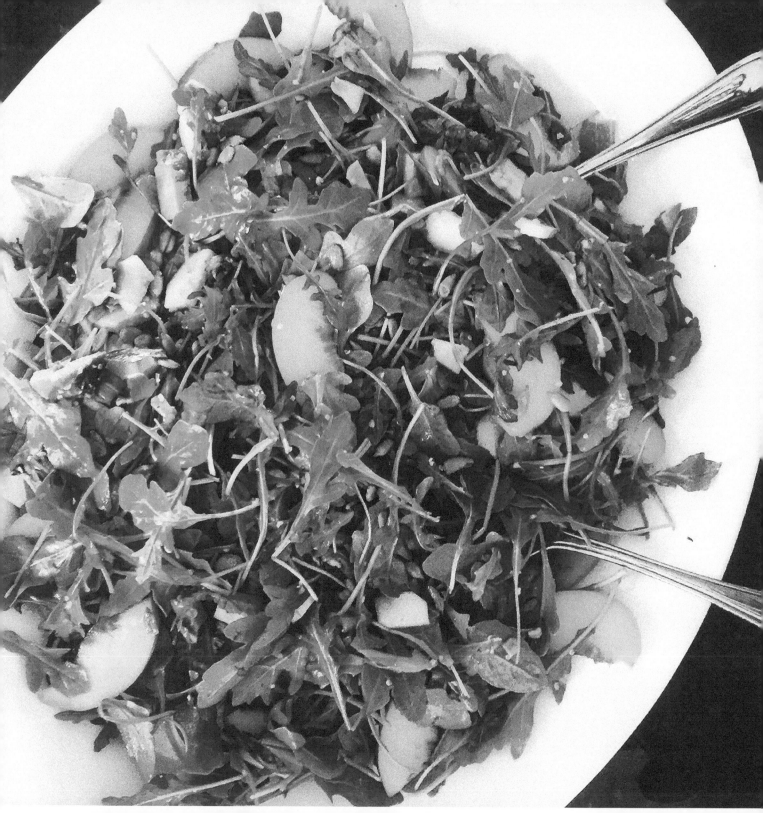

ARUGULA & PEACHES SALAD

This is a great salad for any summer gathering, combining the sweet hint of peach with the tangy arugula leaves. It also makes a beautiful presentation on a table alongside BBQ meat, roasted vegetables, and fresh lemonade.

HERE IS WHAT YOU NEED:

1 bag arugula
   (approximately 6 cups)
2 peaches, sliced thin
½ avocado, diced
1 cucumber, sliced thin
½ cup sunflower seeds

Dressing:
1 lime, juice only
2 tablespoons olive oil
1 tablespoon maple syrup
2 tablespoons hemp seeds
Pinch salt

LET'S DO THIS:

1. Combine the arugula, sunflower seeds, and cucumbers in a large salad bowl or large platter.

2. Mix the dressing and pour over the greens. Toss lightly with your hands.

3. Spread the avocado and peaches and toss lightly again, being careful not to break them.

SUPERFOODS SALAD

This is a casual greens salad with loads of crunch, good fats, and superfoods. Sprouts are packed with nutrients and easy to incorporate into any salad or sandwich. Next time you are at the produce aisle, grab a package of sprouts and toss it into a salad or a sandwich for extra boost of super foods.

HERE IS WHAT YOU NEED:

1 bag arugula (or small box or a bowl full)

1 head radicchio, chopped

1 yellow squash, grated or diced small

1 cup sprouts (any kind), separated

1 avocado, cubed

4-5 tablespoons raw tahini

1 lemon, juice only

Salt and pepper

LET'S DO THIS:

Combine all in a large salad bowl and toss lightly. Bon appétit!

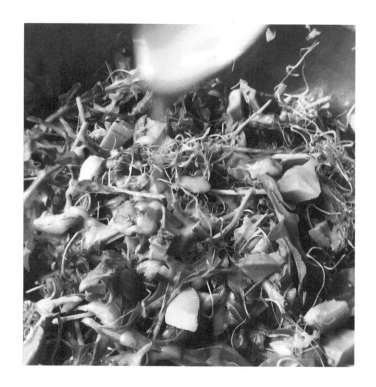

POWERHOUSE SALAD

This colorful and healthy salad is great to keep in the fridge for those moments when you open the fridge in search of something to chew on... your body will thank you! Use the quantities as a guideline, not a blueprint. Add or subtract any of the ingredients as your heart (and taste buds) desire.

HERE IS WHAT YOU NEED:

4 Persian cucumbers
2 large tomatoes, cubed
1 avocado, cubed
1 package lentil sprouts
1 handful raw sunflower seeds
5-6 scallions, chopped small
3 tablespoons olive oil
Salt and pepper
1 lemon, juice only

LET'S DO THIS:

Combine everything in a large salad bowl and toss. Enjoy!

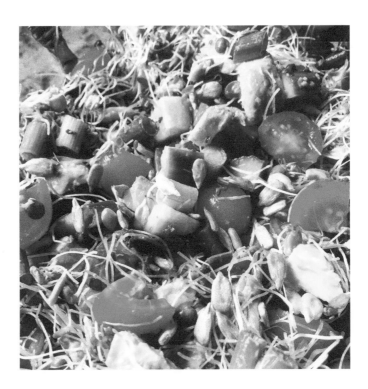

WARM SPINACH SALAD

This warm salad can be a side or a main dish. It is packed with good-for-you flavors and will be sure to leave you satisfied.

HERE IS WHAT YOU NEED:

3 tablespoons coconut oil

1 tablespoon olive oil

2 shallots, diced

½ red onion, diced

1 can organic garbanzo beans, rinsed and drained

1 bag (or 4 handfuls) baby spinach leaves

½ cup sun-dried tomatoes

2 tablespoons apple cider vinegar

½ cup water

Salt and pepper

LET'S DO THIS:

1. Add the coconut oil to a skillet and sauté the shallots and onions. Add the garlic and the garbanzo beans and cook for 3 minutes, then add the sun-dried tomatoes.

2. Season with salt, pepper, apple cider vinegar, and water. Bring to a gentle boil and simmer for a couple of minutes.

3. Turn off the heat and add the spinach. Stir gently to ensure all of the spinach is lightly cooked.

4. Toss well and drizzle 1 tablespoon olive oil on top for extra flavor.

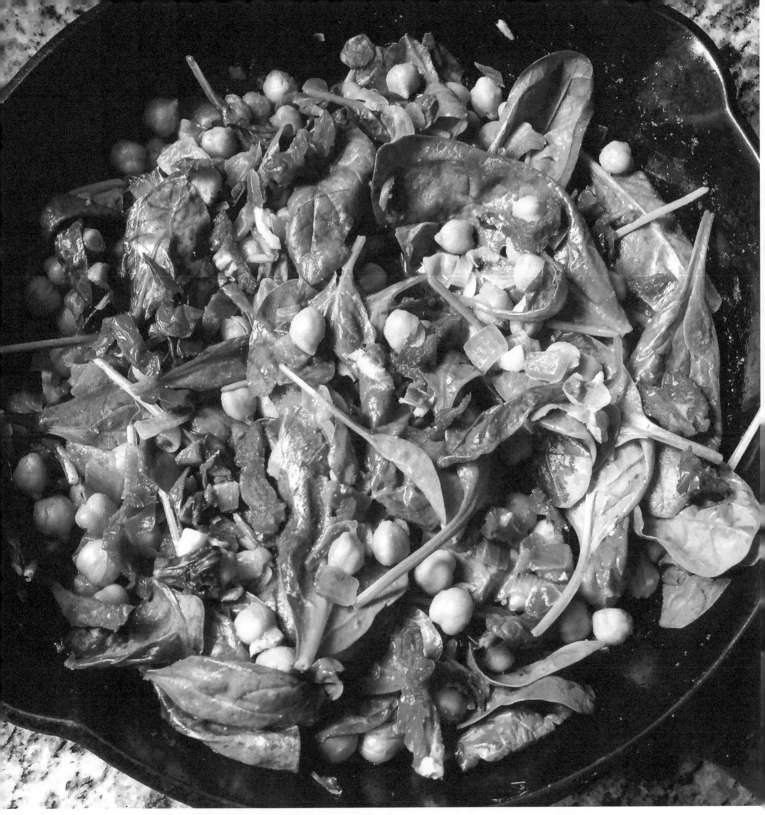

ARUGULA & BUTTERNUT SQUASH SALAD

This beautiful salad steals the show. Its unusual flavors merge surprisingly well. The salad dressing takes a couple of minutes to prepare, but it is worth the effort. This is a great salad for autumn and Thanksgiving, but my family enjoys it year-round.

HERE IS WHAT YOU NEED:

1 bag (or 5 cups) arugula

2 lbs. butternut squash, cubed

4 tablespoons olive oil

1 tablespoon maple syrup

Dressing:

¾ cup water

3 tablespoons maple syrup

3 tablespoons apple cider vinegar

½ red onion, diced small

2 garlic cloves, minced

1 tablespoon Dijon mustard

¼ cup olive oil

LET'S DO THIS:

1. Toss the butternut squash with olive oil and maple syrup and roast at 425°F for 30 minutes. Let it cool.

2. While the butternut squash is roasting, prepare the dressing: In a saucepan, combine the water, maple syrup, apple cider vinegar, chopped onion, and garlic. Bring to a gentle boil, lower the heat and keep cooking for 3-4 minutes. Take off the stove and add the mustard and olive oil. Mix well.

3. Spread the arugula on a large platter, arrange the butternut squash on top, and drizzle the dressing evenly all over and serve.

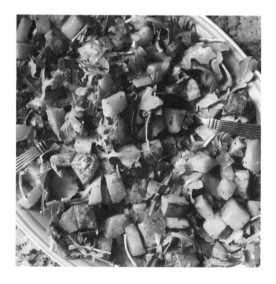

SUPERCHARGED KALE SALAD

All of the ingredients in this salad are packed with super nutrients. It has a nice balance of tangy and somewhat sweet ingredients that go very well together. This salad can be made ahead of time and will last in the refrigerator for at least a couple of days. The Dijon mustard gives it a chock full of flavors, so there is no need for salt and pepper.

HERE IS WHAT YOU NEED:

1 bunch kale, chopped

1 red bell pepper, diced

1 cucumber, diced

1 tablespoon olive oil

1 tablespoon blend of seeds like chia seeds, hemp seeds, flaxseed, or millet

1-2 tablespoons Dijon mustard

3 tablespoons apple cider vinegar

2-3 tablespoons almond slices, for garnish

LET'S DO THIS:

Combine everything in a large salad bowl and toss with two wooden spoons for about 3-4 minutes. Garnish with almonds before serving.

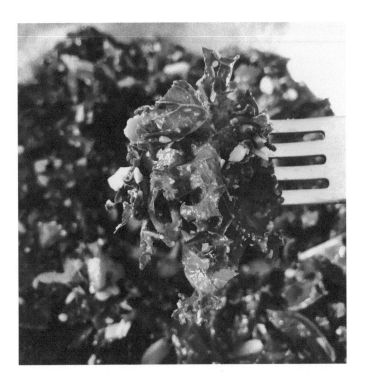

PURPLE CABBAGE & CITRUS SALAD

The beautiful colors of this salad make you dive in and eat it all up! It delivers loads of nutrients and flavors with a great crunch. Typically, I make it in the winter when clementines and oranges are in season, but you can enjoy it year round.

HERE IS WHAT YOU NEED:

3 cups shredded
   purple cabbage

1 carrot, shredded

¼ cup chopped pecans

2 clementines, peeled,
   divided and halved

3 tablespoons apple
   cider vinegar

1 tablespoon maple syrup

1 tablespoon olive oil

LET'S DO THIS:

Combine everything except the clementines in a large salad bowl and toss well using two wooden spoons. Add the clementines at the end and toss lighting to spread them around.

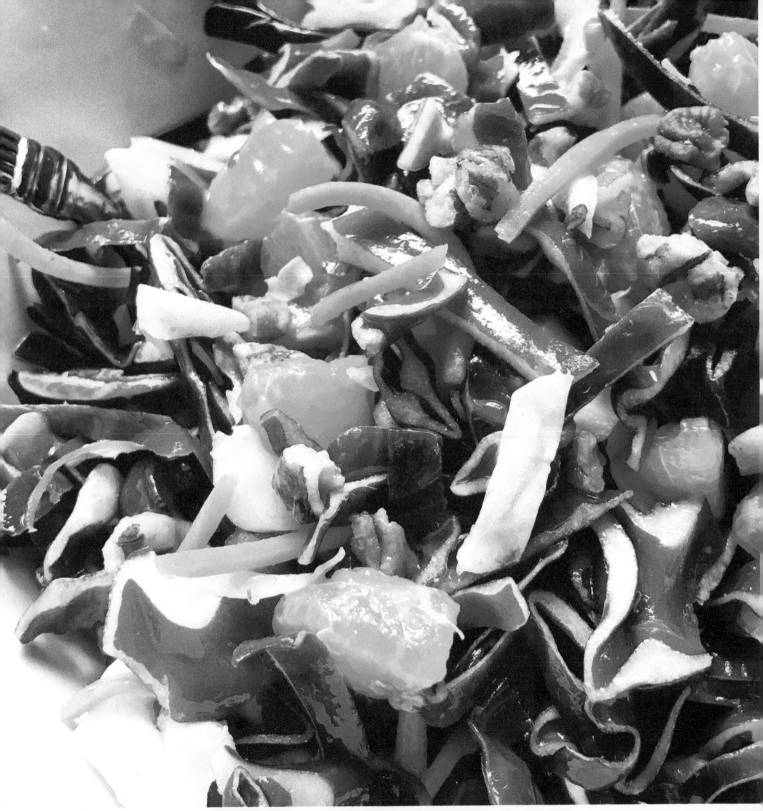

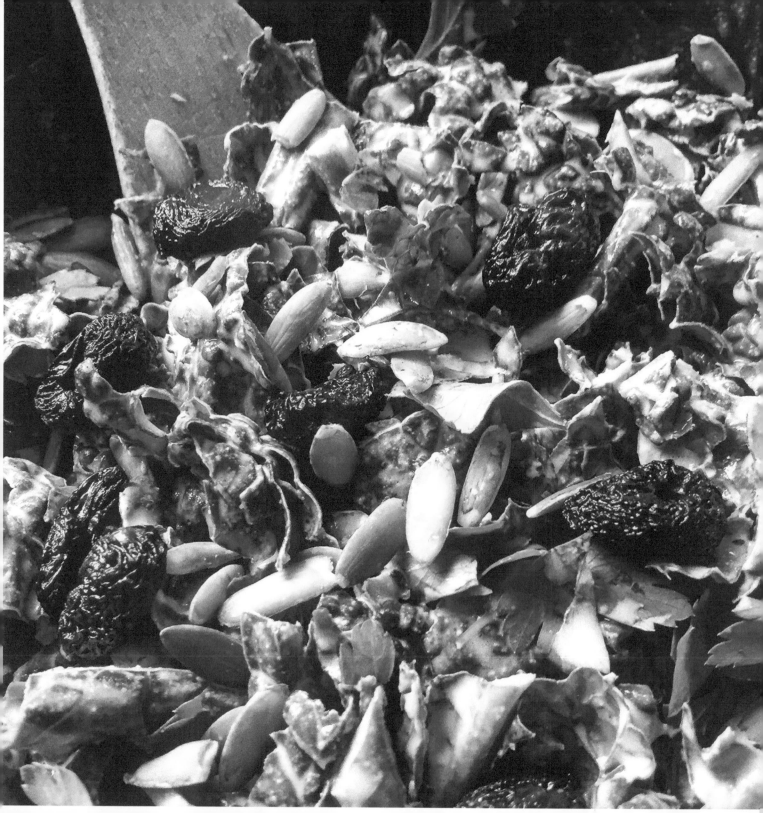

FANCY KALE SALAD

If kale is not your go-to food, this salad might turn you into a kale fanatic. Unlike other leafy greens, kale will keep fresh in the refrigerator for a few days, with its dressing. It will actually taste better and have a better texture than the first day. Try it and enjoy the convenience of a salad you can prepare ahead of time!

HERE IS WHAT YOU NEED:

1 bunch kale, chopped small

1 cup chopped parsley

¼ cup pumpkin seed

1 handful dried sour cherries, cut in halves

Dressing:

½ cup raw tahini

½ cup water

1 lemon, juice only

1 tablespoon maple syrup

Salt and pepper

Mix well in a small bowl with a fork

LET'S DO THIS:

1. Combine the kale and parsley in a large bowl.

2. Drizzle the dressing over the kale. Using two wooden spoons, work the dressing into the kale for a few minutes.

3. Sprinkle the pumpkin seeds and tart cherries on top. Enjoy!

VERY BERRY GREENS SALAD

This refreshing salad is a great companion to a summer BBQ dinner or as a stand alone satisfying lunch. It is packed with antioxidants and superfoods to boost immunity and energy. Enjoy!

HERE IS WHAT YOU NEED:

A bowl of mixed greens like kale, arugula, baby spinach, etc.

1 green apple, diced

1 avocado, diced

½ cup chopped pecans

1 cup fresh raspberries or blueberries

Dressing:

2 tablespoons avocado or olive oil

2 tablespoons balsamic vinegar

1 tablespoon maple syrup or honey

1 tablespoon red wine vinegar

LET'S DO THIS:

Combine everything except for the berries in a large salad bowl and toss lightly just enough to coat the greens with the dressing. Sprinkle the berries before serving.

Seeds for Thought... *What's better, Non-GMO or Organic? Choose organic whenever possible since organic foods guaranteed to be synthetic pesticides free, and they are always non-GMO.*

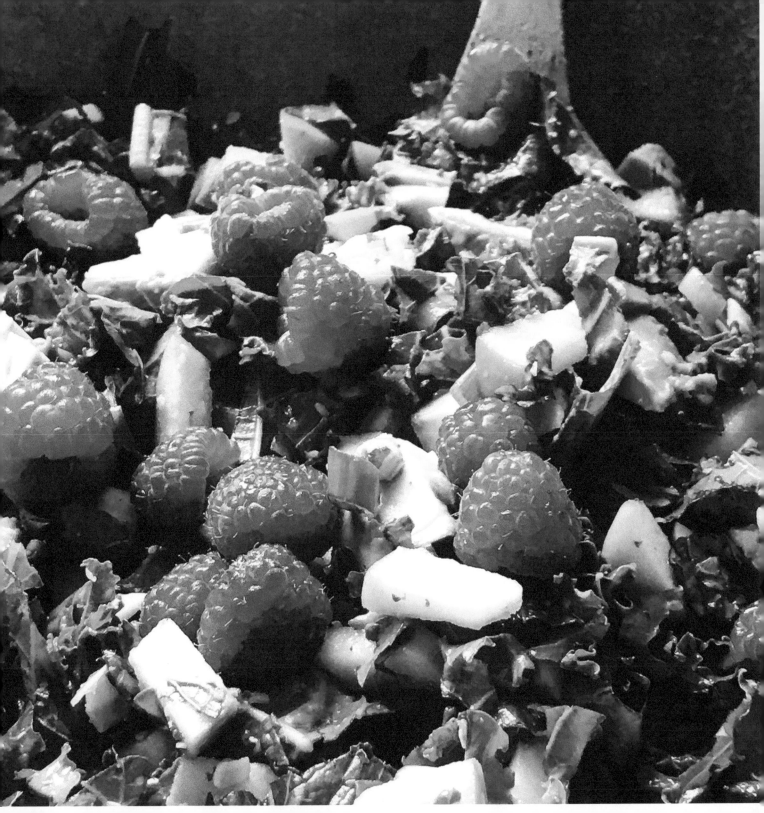

RADISH MEDLEY

This colorful salad is easy to prepare, light, crunchy, and oh-so-good-for-you!

HERE IS WHAT YOU NEED:

1 bunch (or 3 cups)
  radishes, chopped

2 celery stalks, chopped

Handful of walnuts
  or pecans, chopped

1 apple, cubed

½ cup chopped parsley

Dressing:

3 tablespoons olive oil

1 lime (or lemon), juice only

Salt and pepper

LET'S DO THIS:

Combine all in a small bowl and toss well.

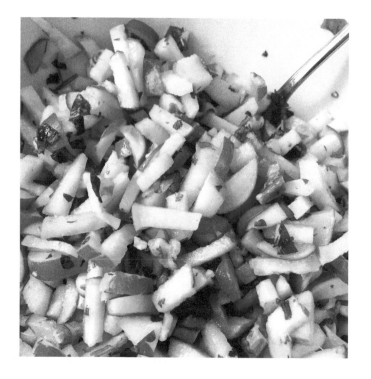

MOROCCAN CARROT SALAD

Carrots are normally used as minor addition to a dish or a soup. Here, carrots have the starring role, beautiful, tasty, and of course, incredibly nutritious. This dish can be eaten as a salad or atop a bed of mixed greens, with a drizzle of tahini sauce on top. It is great to keep in the fridge, even as a snack.

HERE IS WHAT YOU NEED:

4-5 lbs. carrots, peeled and cut to ¼"-½" discs (orange or tri-color carrots can be used)

Dressing:

¼ cup extra virgin olive oil

1 tablespoon cumin

½ teaspoon garlic powder

¼ teaspoon chili powder

3 garlic cloves, minced

Salt and pepper

Handful parsley, chopped

LET'S DO THIS:

1. Cook the carrots in a pot with water. Bring to a boil and cook for 20 minutes. They should be cooked al dente; with a firm bite and not too soft.

2. Drain the carrots and let them cool. Transfer to a bowl and add the rest of the ingredients.

3. Toss well and store in a jar in the refrigerator up to a week.

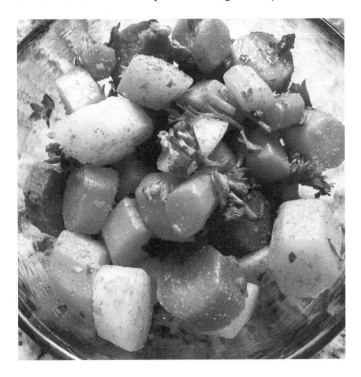

LIFE OF THE PARTY GUACAMOLE

Avocados are a treasure trove of nutrients and healthy fats. They are naturally delicious fruit you can enjoy daily, on a toast or salad, or even by itself with a pinch of sea salt. This is an easy recipe for homemade guac everyone will love to dig into, either with tortilla chips or cut-up vegetables.

HERE IS WHAT YOU NEED:

3-4 ripe avocados

1 medium onion (red or white), diced small

1 jalapeno, diced small

1 tomato, diced small

1 cup cilantro or parsley, chopped well

2 garlic cloves, minced

One lime (or lemon), juice only

Salt and pepper

Pinch of chili powder (optional)

LET'S DO THIS:

Combine everything in a bowl and mix gently with a spoon. The mixture should be chunky, perfect for scooping up with a carrot stick or tortilla chip. It's party time!

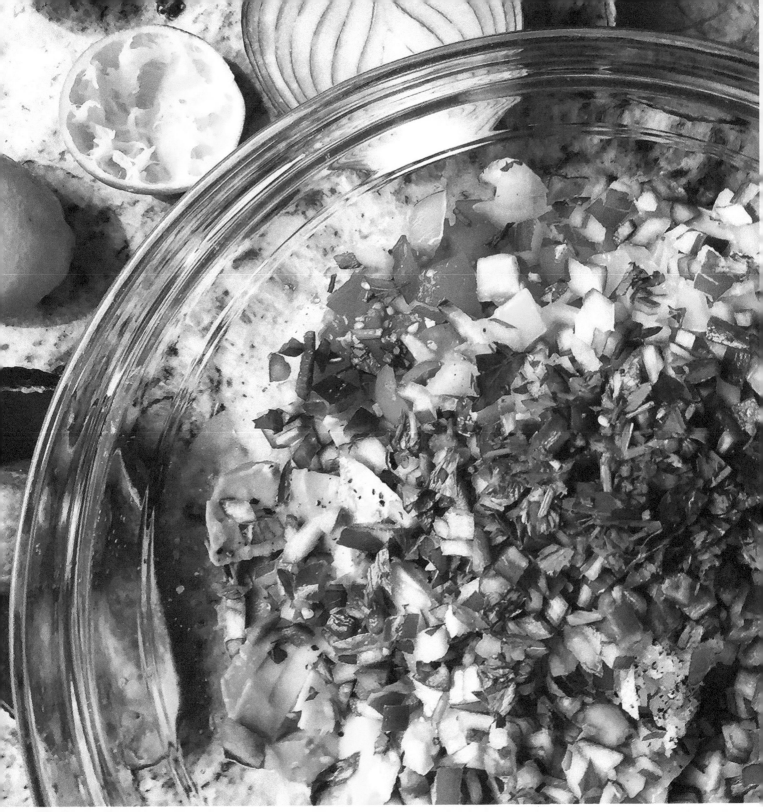

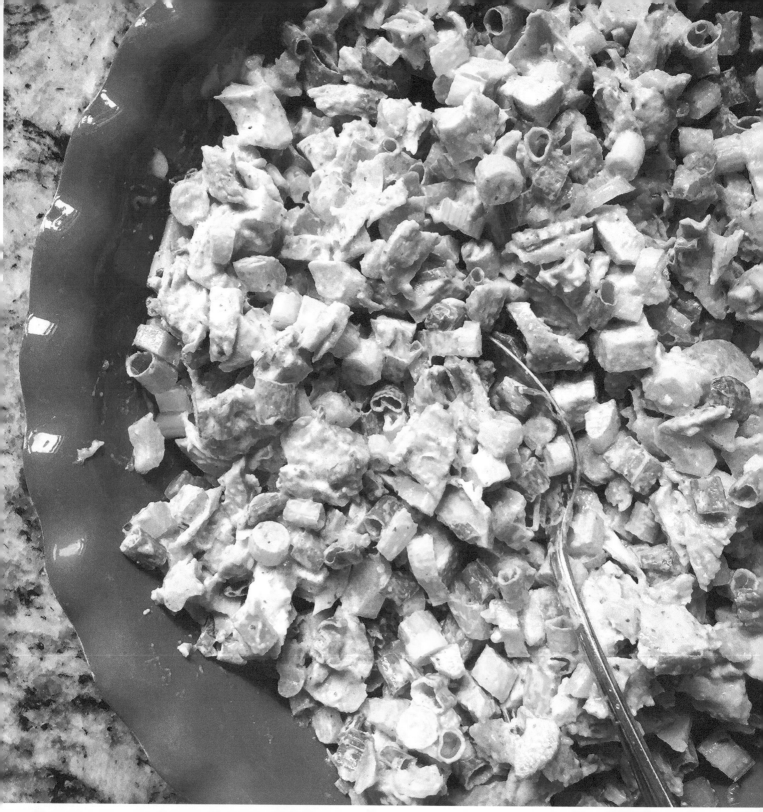

AUTHENTIC CHICKEN SALAD

There's nothing like a homemade chicken salad! The best-tasting chicken for a salad comes from either a homemade chicken soup or roasted chicken leftovers. If you want to save time, take the meat off the bones with your hands, it might be messy, but worth the effort!

HERE IS WHAT YOU NEED:

2-3 cups chicken meat, diced (no bones or skin)

5-6 scallions, diced

1 onion, diced (red or white onion)

2-3 celery stalks, diced small

2 tablespoons organic mayonnaise

1 tablespoon Dijon mustard

Salt and pepper

LET'S DO THIS:

Mix all of the ingredients in a bowl until they are incorporated evenly. Refrigerate and use within 4-5 days.

Optional:

- Add 1 teaspoon turmeric or cumin to switch up the flavor and color.

- Scoop the salad over greens and pack it up for lunch.

- Add the juice from half a lemon.

- Use romaine lettuce or collard greens as flatbreads to roll up the chicken salad. Serve the wraps for lunch or dinner with side toppings like diced tomatoes or sprouts.

- Add diced boiled eggs or roasted potatoes.

STRAWBERRY FIELDS SALAD

This is a fabulous salad that pairs well with any meal. It is fresh, light and makes a beautiful presentation. If you don't like kale, substitute with any other greens such as arugula, baby spinach, or mixed lettuce.

HERE IS WHAT YOU NEED:

1 bunch kale, chopped into bite-size pieces (or about 6 cups of any other greens)

2 cups sliced strawberries

1 cup cooked red quinoa

Dressing:

½ red onion, diced small

3 tablespoons olive oil

2 tablespoons red wine vinegar

2 tablespoons honey or maple syrup

Salt and pepper

LET'S DO THIS:

1. Mix the dressing in a jar and let sit for 10 minutes.

1. Combine the kale and the quinoa in a salad bowl and toss with the dressing for a couple of minutes.

2. Add the strawberries and toss lightly one more time. Serve!

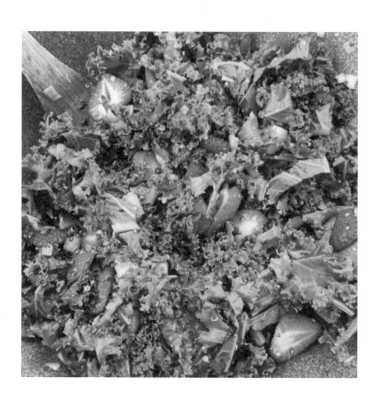

BERRY TANGY BEET SALAD

This salad is bursting with flavors and colors, thanks to the beets, carrots, dried sour cherries, and cranberries. It's a good dish to have in the fridge for those moments when you need a crunch without the guilt or to bring to a potluck party.

HERE IS WHAT YOU NEED:

4-5 beets, boiled in water until softened

2-3 carrots, cut into thin sticks

⅓ cup dried sour cherries

⅓ cup dried cranberries

1 lemon, juice only

3 tablespoons olive oil

Dash salt

⅓ cup chopped pecans

LET'S DO THIS:

1. Dice the beets into about ¼" size pieces.

2. Add all the ingredients except the pecans in a bowl and toss well.

3. Sprinkle the pecans on top.

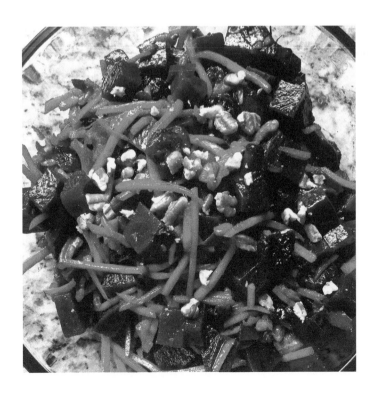

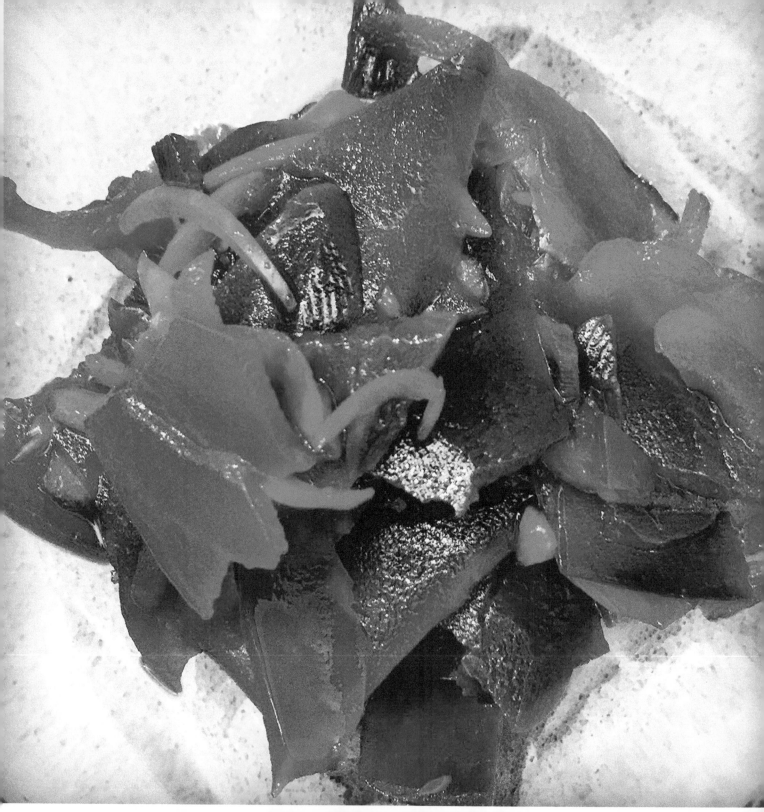

SAVORY BEETS SALAD

This is a great side salad for entertaining or to keep in the fridge as a healthy snack. It will add a pop of color to your table as well as a plate full of nutrients. The dressing transforms the bland beets into a delicious and flavorful vegetable.

HERE IS WHAT YOU NEED:

5 whole beets, boiled in water until softened

1 onion, slivered

2 tablespoons olive oil

3 tablespoons apple cider vinegar

3 tablespoons water

½ lemon, juice only

1 tablespoon honey or maple syrup

Salt

LET'S DO THIS:

1. Slice the beets thinly then add them to a bowl with the onions.

2. Mix the dressing well and pour it over the beet mixture. Toss well.

3. Store in an airtight container in the refrigerator until ready to serve. It will keep well in the fridge up to a week.

CUCUMBER & MINT SALAD

This salad is perfect for the summer months when crunchy cucumbers are on every produce stand. Any kind of cucumbers will deliver good results as long as they are fresh and crunchy. It pairs well with grilled meat or chicken or on top of a pile of greens for lunch.

HERE IS WHAT YOU NEED:

4 medium cucumbers, diced into small cubes

Handful chopped mint leaves

Dressing:

1 tablespoon olive oil

1 teaspoon maple syrup

3 tablespoons apple cider vinegar

3 tablespoons water

1 tablespoon hemp seeds (optional)

LET'S DO THIS:

1. Combine the dressing ingredients and mix well in a small jar.

2. Combine everything else in a medium salad bowl and toss gently with the dressing.

3. Garnish with fresh mint leaves.

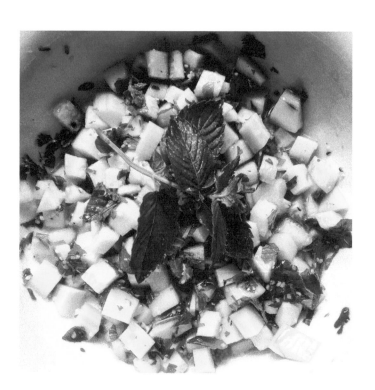

KALE & MANGO SALAD WITH AVOCADO DRESSING

This salad is delicious! The creamy avocado dressing just about dances with the light sweetness of the mango. This salad makes a beautiful presentation on the table whether you are entertaining or taking it with you to a party.

HERE IS WHAT YOU NEED:

1 bunch kale, chopped into bite-size pieces

2 cups diced mango

3 tablespoons shelled hemp seeds (optional)

Dressing:

1 avocado

½ small onion

½ lemon, juice only

1 tablespoon apple cider vinegar

Salt and pepper

1 cup cilantro (or parsley)

2 tablespoons olive oil

1 garlic clove

LET'S DO THIS:

1. In a food processor, combine the dressing ingredients and process until smooth and creamy. If it is too thick, add lemon juice or oil.

2. Place the kale in a large salad bowl. Add the dressing and toss for a couple of minutes.

3. Add the mangos and toss lightly. Sprinkle with shelled hemp seeds before serving.

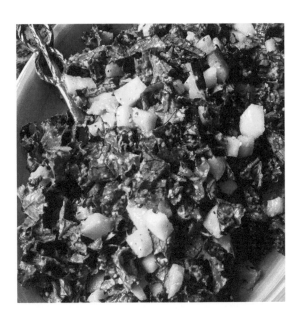

ROBUST KALE SALAD

This vibrant, high-flavor salad is suitable for any festive meal as a side dish or as the main course. The pecans, cranberries and kale compliment each other perfectly with the right amount of crunch and flavors! You will not have any leftovers of this one. The kale can be substituted with baby spinach leaves.

HERE IS WHAT YOU NEED:

1 bunch kale, chopped into bite-size pieces

2 cups purple cabbage, chopped

1 cup dried cranberries

½ cup chopped pecans

Dressing:

¼ cup olive oil

2 tablespoons apple cider vinegar

1 tablespoon maple syrup

1 heaping teaspoon cumin

Pinch salt

LET'S DO THIS:

1. Mix the dressing well in a jar.

2. Combine everything in a large salad bowl. Toss with the dressing for a couple of minutes with two wooden spoons. Note: If you are using spinach instead of kale, pour the dressing just before serving.

Seeds for Thought... Most dried fruits have sugar and sometimes oil added to them in the manufacturing process. Read the label and make sure your dried fruits contain fruits only.

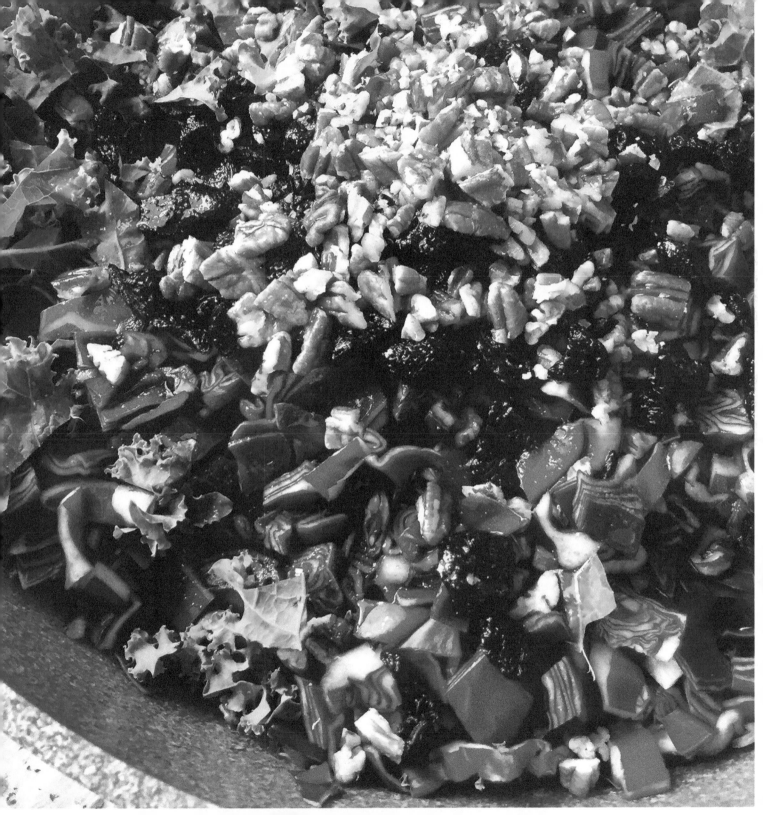

QUICK QUINOA SALAD

Packed with protein and fiber, quinoa is a superfood that can taste a little bland and boring by itself. Here is a quick, colorful, and flavorful way to jazz up your quinoa into a flavorful and satisfying salad for any time, any season.

HERE IS WHAT YOU NEED:

2 cups cooked quinoa (use instructions on the back of the package)

1 jar (12-oz.) roasted peppers, chopped small

1 English cucumber, cubed small

3 cups baby spinach, chopped into small, bite-size pieces

3 tablespoons olive oil

1 lemon, juice only

Salt and pepper

LET'S DO THIS:

Combine all the ingredients in a large salad bowl and toss well.

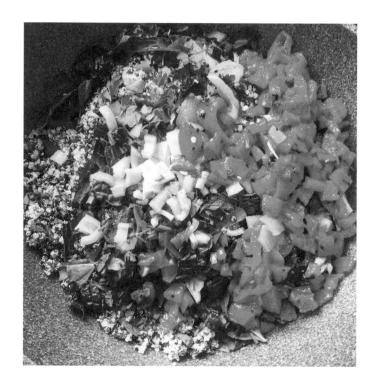

BRIGHT BROCCOLI SALAD

I have a confession to make... I don't like broccoli! But since it is one of the most nutrient-packed vegetables out there, I have learned to like it. My two favorite ways to eat broccoli are roasted or tossed in a crunchy salad, as is the case here. This concert of flavors—the broccoli, cashews and roasted red peppers—is so delicious, everyone will ask for more.

HERE IS WHAT YOU NEED:

- 1 head broccoli, chopped into small florets, about ½"
- 2 roasted red peppers (from a jar is ok)
- 2 handfuls cashew pieces

Dressing:

- ½ cup mayonnaise (preferred organic or homemade)
- 1 tablespoon honey
- 2 tablespoons apple cider vinegar

LET'S DO THIS:

1. In a large bowl combine the broccoli, peppers and cashews.

2. In a small bowl mix the dressing and pour it over the broccoli and toss for a couple of minutes to make sure everything is coated evenly.

3. Garnish with chopped roasted pepper and cashew pieces.

4. Can be served immediately or made a few hours ahead.

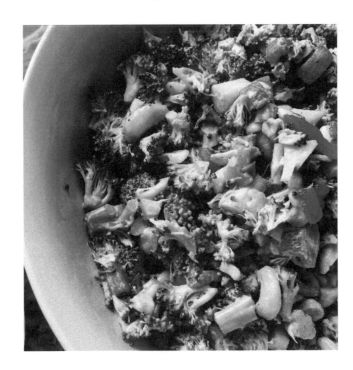

WATERMELON & ARUGULA SALAD

This salad will steal the show at any cookout! It goes well with any BBQ foods and will decorate the dinner table beautifully.

HERE IS WHAT YOU NEED:

½ small watermelon, cut into 3/4" cubes

6 cups fresh arugula

½ cup chopped mint leaves

4 tablespoon full-fat goat cheese, crumbled (or more)

½ red onion, chopped small (optional)

Dressing:

3 tablespoons olive oil

2 tablespoons red wine vinegar

1 tablespoon maple syrup

Salt and pepper

LET'S DO THIS:

1. Combine the watermelon, arugula, mint leaves and onion in a large salad bowl or a large platter.

2. Mix the dressing in a jar and drizzle all over the salad a few minutes before serving. Toss gently so the watermelon doesn't get too watery.

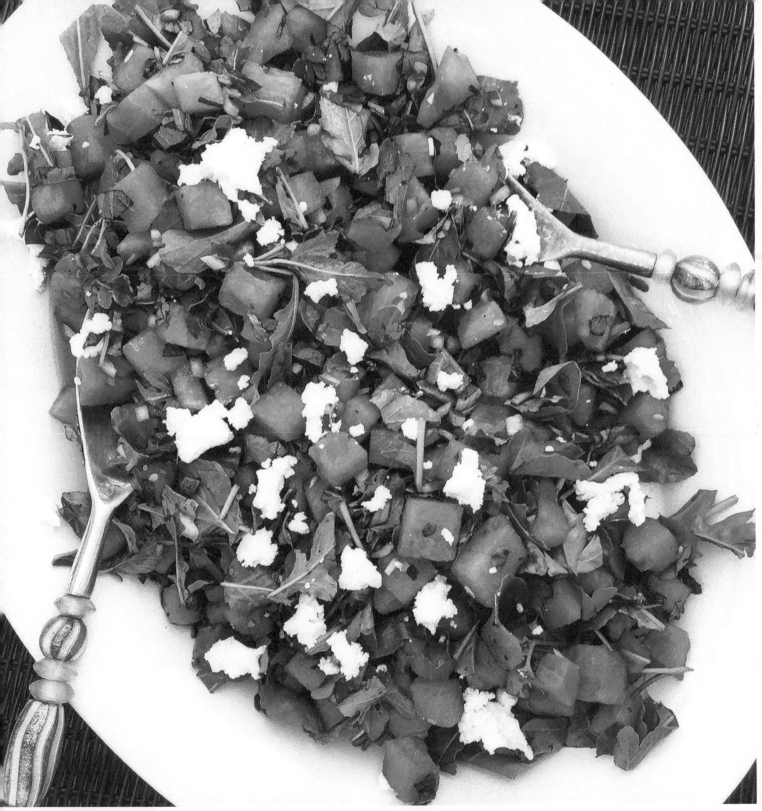

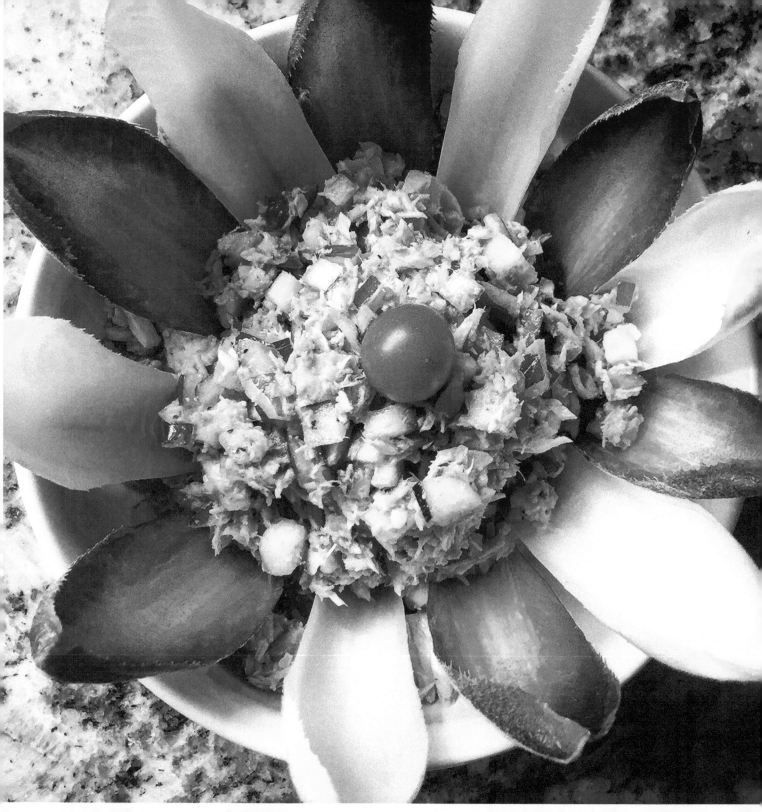

TRUE TUNA SALAD

Tuna salad can be healthy and delicious, especially when it is homemade. It is very easy to make at home, even in a large quantity, and you can enjoy it for a couple of days as a healthful snack or pack for lunch in a lettuce wrap. This version of tuna salad is clean of fillers, sugars, and chemicals, so you can enjoy it by the bowl full!

HERE IS WHAT YOU NEED:

4 cans high-quality tuna
(2 packed in olive oil, 2
in water)

1 large cucumber, diced small

1 red onion, diced small

1 celery stem, diced small

2 tablespoons olive oil

½ teaspoon turmeric

Salt and pepper
(taste before adding salt)

Endive leaves, for serving
(optional)

LET'S DO THIS:

1. Combine all the ingredients in a bowl and mix well, breaking the big tuna chunks to smaller pieces.

2. Optional: Serve in the center of a ring of endive leaves (see left), for a pretty presentation.

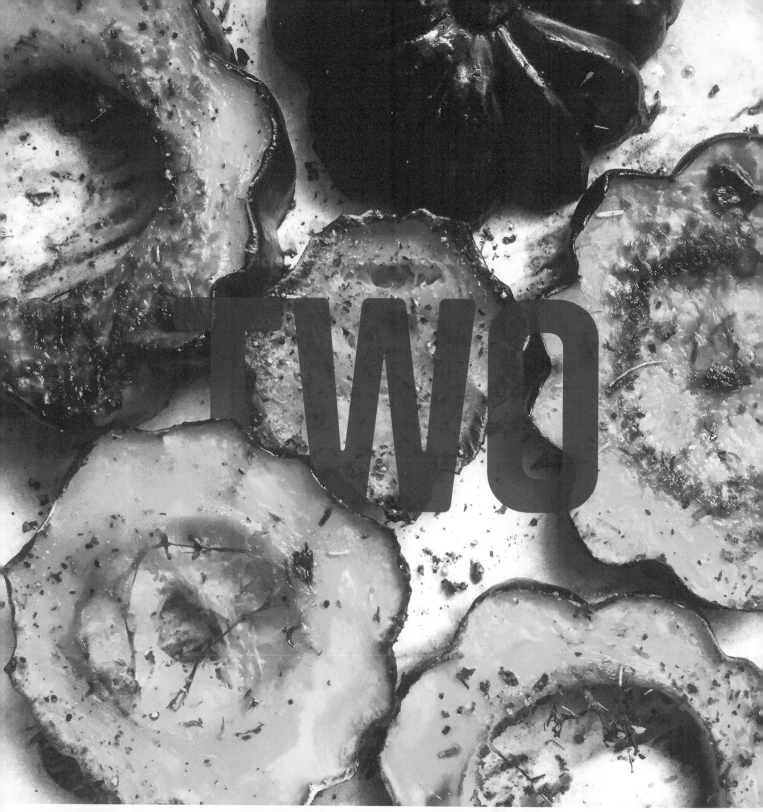

VEGETABLES
Rule!

71

Vegetables are truly a gift of nature: eating an assortment of fruits and vegetables will supply nearly all the nutrients we need. Strive to eat mostly vegetables and other plant-based foods and you will be on the right path for a healthy lifestyle. There are so many ways to cook vegetables, from frying to boiling to roasting or simply toss them raw in salads. They transform easily with just a few simple herbs and spices so you don't even have to work hard to enjoy their beauty and great taste. Make sure you rotate ingredients and cooking methods to get an assortment of vitamins and nutrients. Fill up your cart with seasonal and colorful vegetables and use these recipes for inspiration. But most importantly, have fun with it!

COLORFUL ROASTED VEGETABLE PLATTER

This platter is always a great addition to any meal, festive or casual; everyone loves at least one ingredient, so it is a good option for entertaining a large crowd. Select colorful vegetables and arrange them in sections to make a stunning presentation.

If you are using a few kinds of vegetables at a time, it is a good idea to separate them on a baking sheet since their cooking times vary. This way it is easier to take them out of the oven when they are ready and let the other vegetables roast until they are done. Also, roasting them separately gives you the option to season each one differently.

Leftovers roasted vegetables are always a blessing, as they keep very well in the refrigerator and can be used for a few days after as salad toppers, sandwiches, or incorporated in a colorful frittata.

HOW TO ROAST VEGETABLES:

Select 4-8 varieties, such as sweet potatoes, cauliflower florets, beets, bell peppers, asparagus, garlic, purple onions, Brussels sprouts, broccoli, yellow potatoes, and mushrooms. Make sure you have an assortment of colors for an eye-catching presentation.

Clean, cut into chunks and pat them dry with paper towels. Drying them is a crucial step to ensure the vegetables are not soggy. Toss each type of vegetable in either olive oil or coconut oil (use refined coconut oil to avoid an overpowering coconut flavor). Season each vegetable with your favorite seasoning. Some ideas include Salt and pepper, turmeric, cumin, paprika, dried or fresh thyme / rosemary / sage / oregano. However, sea salt and pepper are always the best choices, and you can't go wrong using just those two.

Arrange the vegetables in groups on a baking sheet lined with parchment paper or foil. Use two baking sheets if it's too crowded so that the hot air can circulate each vegetable. Roast at 425°F for about half an hour, then keep checking every few minutes to make sure they are done and not over- or under-cooked. Usually, the potatoes, beets, Brussels sprouts, and carrots will take longer to roast, about 45 minutes. Other vegetables like asparagus, cauliflower, peppers, mushrooms, and onions take about 30-35 minutes.

Arrange the vegetables on a large platter and serve warm or at room temperature.

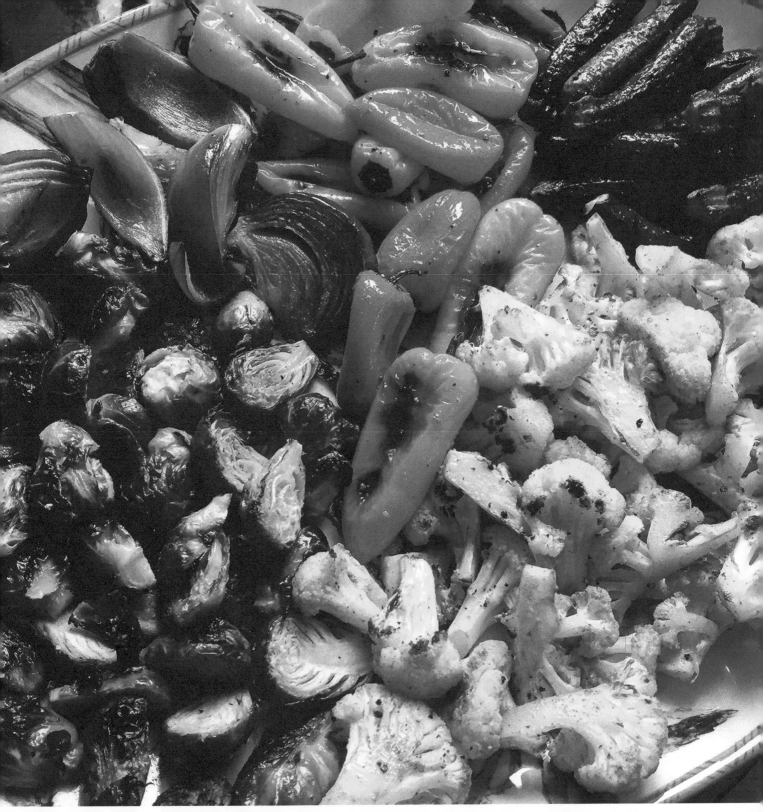

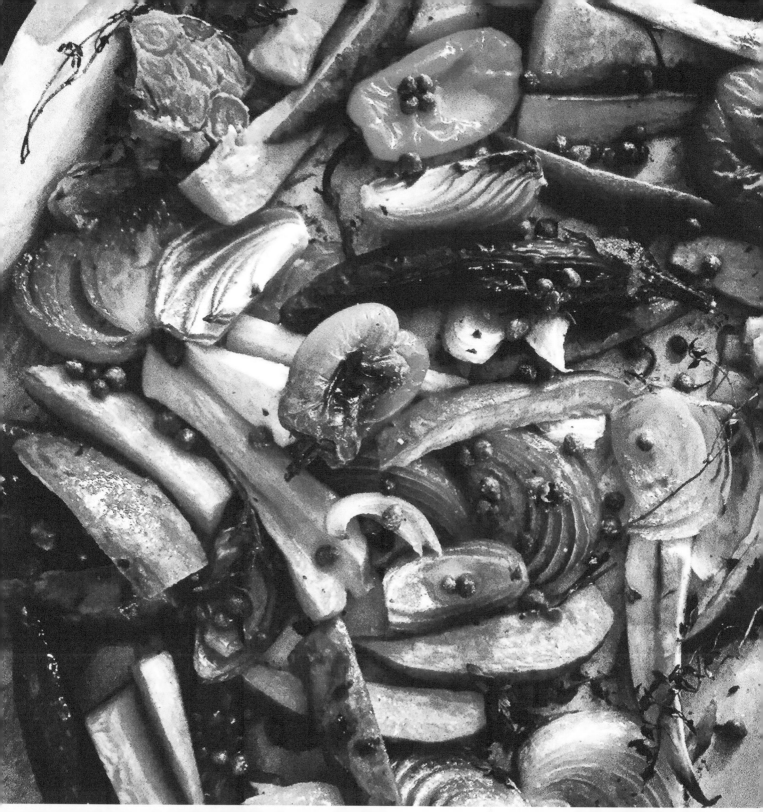

FANCY ROASTED VEGETABLES

This recipe is a fabulous display of fall root vegetables, paired with a contrasting light and tangy dressing.

HERE IS WHAT YOU NEED:

4 sweet potatoes, sliced into wedges

3 parsnips, sliced into wedges

2 purple onion, quartered

2 white onion, quartered

2 garlic heads, cut in half

6 mini peppers or other bell peppers (keep the stem on)

3 mini eggplants, halved (stem on)

5 sprigs rosemary

5 sprigs thyme

¼ cup olive oil

Salt and pepper

Dressing:

1 lemon, juice only

3 tablespoons capers (rinsed)

1 tablespoon maple syrup

1 tablespoon Dijon mustard

LET'S DO THIS:

1. Prepare the vegetables by cleaning them and patting them dry. In a large bowl, toss the vegetables with the oil, salt and pepper.

2. Arrange them on a flat roasting pan lined with parchment paper and roast at 425°F for 45 minutes or until the edges of the vegetables are golden brown.

3. In the meantime, mix the dressing in a small bowl. Drizzle all over the vegetables, once they get out of the oven.

CARROT SOUFFLÉ

This is a traditional and timeless dish we enjoy in every special holiday meal. It is a delicious sweet side dish that compliments any chicken and meat dishes very well. I have converted the traditional recipe to a healthier version without compromising the taste.

HERE IS WHAT YOU NEED:

2 lbs. carrots, cleaned and cut into chunks

⅓ cup coconut oil

¼ cup coconut sugar

2 heaping tablespoons arrowroot flour or potato starch

¼ teaspoon baking powder

¼ teaspoon baking soda

5 eggs

Topping:

½ cup chopped pecans

⅓ cup coconut sugar

¼ cup melted coconut oil or butter

¼ teaspoon cinnamon

LET'S DO THIS:

1. Place the carrots in a pot with water and bring to a boil. Lower the heat and continue cooking for about 20 minutes, until the carrots are soft to the touch of a sharp knife. Drain and let cool.

2. In the bowl of a food processor, combine the remaining ingredients with the carrots. Process well.

3. Grease an oven-safe dish (about 8"x13") with coconut oil and pour in the carrot mixture. Bake at 375°F for 30 min.

4. In the meantime, mix the topping ingredients together in a small bowl.

5. After the soufflé has baked for 30 minutes, remove the dish from the oven and spread the topping on evenly, then bake for another 15 minutes.

6. Serve right away or prepare a day or two ahead. If making ahead, bake for 30 minutes without the topping, then let the soufflé cool and refrigerate. When you are near ready to serve, add the topping and warm the entire dish in a 350°F oven for 20 minutes.

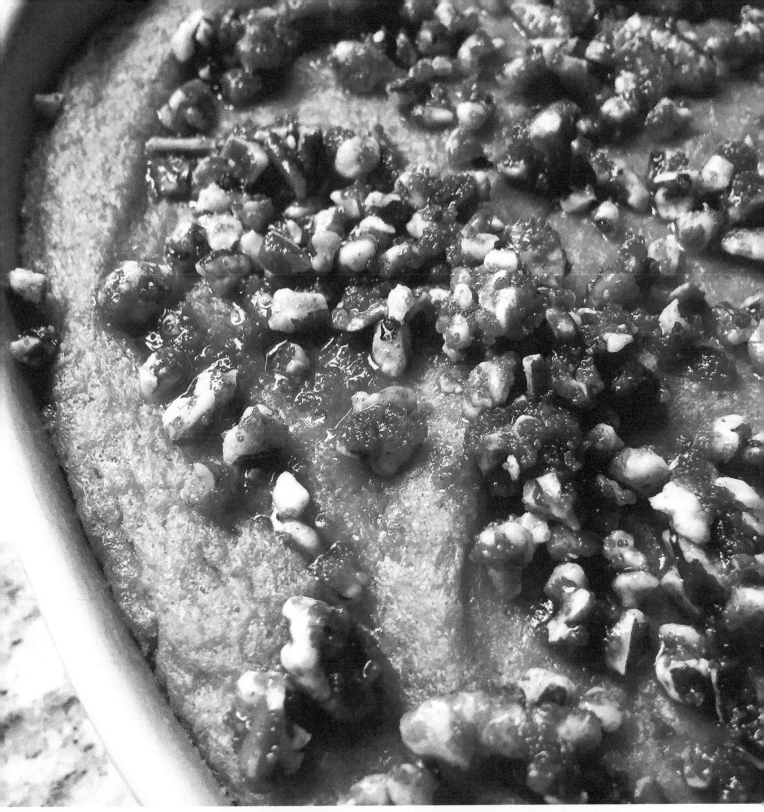

ROMANESCO BROCCOLI

This simple dish is equal parts pretty, flavorful, and healthy. If you can't find Romanesco Broccoli, this recipe will still work well using regular cauliflower.

HERE IS WHAT YOU NEED:

1 head Romanesco Broccoli

Sauce:

1 jar roasted peppers, drained (unflavored)

3 tablespoons capers, rinsed

2 garlic cloves

¼ cup olive oil

Black pepper

LET'S DO THIS:

1. Boil the head of Romanesco in a pot full of water for 20 minutes.

2. While boiling, prepare the sauce in a food processor. Taste and adjust the seasonings as needed.

3. Drain the broccoli, place it in the middle of a baking dish, and spread the sauce all over it. Bake at 375°F for 40 minutes or until the top of the sauce starts to brown.

4. Serve warm and cut as you would for a round cake, or use a big spoon to scoop individual portions onto plates.

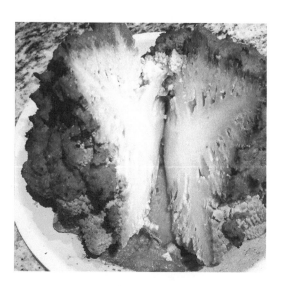

CAULIFLOWER BAKE

Either cauliflower can be used in this recipe, but the purple cauliflower rocks the house in terms of presentation. This dish is very easy to make and yet another fun way to introduce another vegetable on the dinner table.

HERE IS WHAT YOU NEED:

1 head cauliflower (any color)

Dressing:

½ cup organic or homemade mayonnaise

½ cup organic ketchup (or 2 tablespoon organic tomato paste mixed with ½ cup water)

1-2 minced garlic cloves

Salt and pepper (if using ketchup, add less salt)

2 pickles, chopped

LET'S DO THIS:

1. Boil the cauliflower in a pot full of water for about 20-25 minutes, until it softens

2. While the cauliflower is boiling, combine the dressing ingredients and mix well with a spoon.

3. Drain the cauliflower and place it in a middle of a baking dish. Pour the dressing over the head of cauliflower and let it drip down so it almost covers the whole head.

4. Bake at 375°F for 30-40 minutes or until the sauce turns darker roasted color.

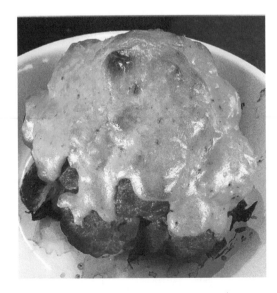

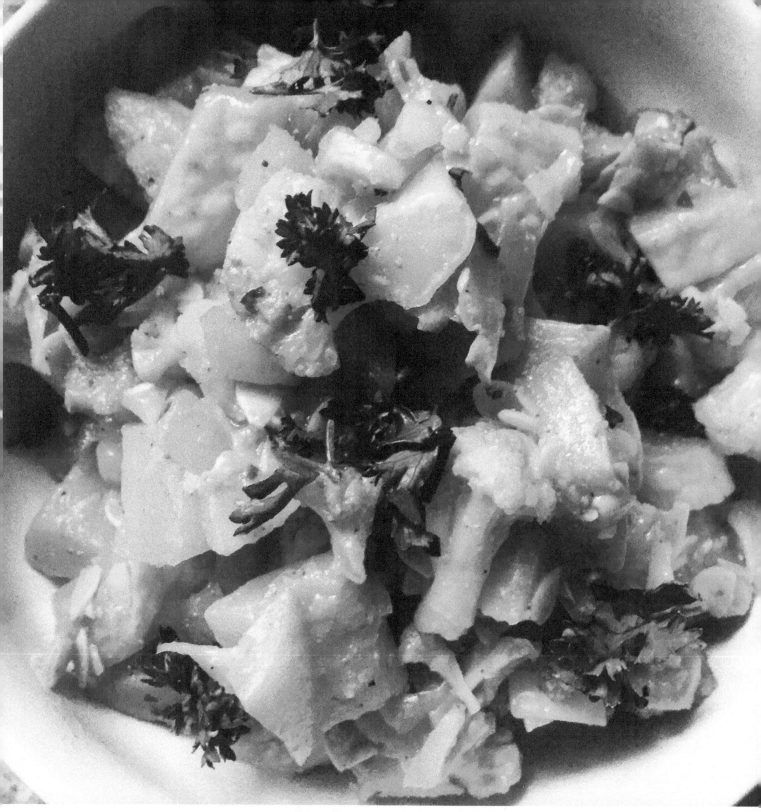

CAULIFLOWER CURRY

This is an Indian inspired dish, showcasing the vibrant colors and rich flavors of this cuisine. Some of the typical Indian spices such as turmeric, curry, and cumin are believed to have anti-inflammatory, and anti-oxidant properties. Here is a simple way to enjoy the many benefits of Indian food.

HERE IS WHAT YOU NEED:

4 tablespoons coconut oil

1 onion, chopped medium

3 medium yellow squash, cubed

1 cauliflower head, cut into small florets

2 garlic cloves, minced

1 teaspoon curry

1 teaspoon turmeric

1 teaspoon garlic powder

1 teaspoon cumin

½ cup water

Salt and pepper

½ cup chopped parsley

LET'S DO THIS:

1. In a medium size pot, heat the coconut oil on medium heat. Add the onions, squash and cauliflower with enough time to sauté in between.

2. Add water and seasonings. Stir gently. Cook on medium heat until it starts boiling. Lower the heat, cover the pot, and simmer for 30-45 minutes. Sprinkle chopped parsley before serving.

3. To enhance the Indian meal experience, serve the curry on top of basmati white rice cooked with aromatic spices like cinnamon and whole cloves. Use one cinnamon stick and 4 cloves per cup of dry rice.

PERFECTLY ROASTED CAULIFLOWER

Once you start munching on these, you can't stop (and why should you?)! It's a simple dish with lots to offer.

HERE IS WHAT YOU NEED:

1 head cauliflower,
    cut into small florets

3 tablespoons coconut
    oil, melted

1 teaspoon sea salt

Freshly ground pepper

½ teaspoon turmeric

LET'S DO THIS:

1. In a large mixing bowl, combine the cauliflower, oil and seasonings. Using two wide wooden spoons, toss everything together for a couple of minutes, until the cauliflower is evenly coated.

2. Spread the cauliflower evenly on a cookie sheet lined with parchment paper, making sure it's not overly crowded and the florets lay flat on the cookie sheet. Roast at 425°F for 40 minutes or until the edges of the cauliflower begin to turn brown.

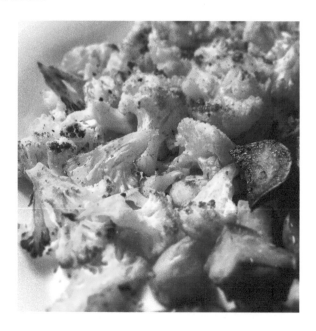

OKRA STEW

This is a traditional dish from my childhood. The climate in Israel is perfect for growing okra, so it is a popular item in the local cuisine. I still remember my grandmother preparing this dish, from shopping for the okra and carefully selecting the pods at the produce stand to cleaning it at home by removing the stem and tip. Lucky us, nowadays, we can find organic, clean, and ready-to-cook okra in the frozen foods section of many grocery stores! Okra is packed with nutrients and healing properties for the digestive system.

HERE IS WHAT YOU NEED:

2 bags frozen okra

1 onion, chopped

2 garlic cloves, crushed

2 tablespoons coconut or olive oil

1 can (14.5oz) stewed organic cubed tomatoes

1 lemon, juice only

Salt and pepper

LET'S DO THIS:

1. In a medium pot (with a lid to be used later in the recipe,) sauté the onions in oil until golden.

2. Add the garlic and sauté lightly. Add the okra and keep sautéing for another 10 minutes. Add the tomatoes, salt and pepper, and lemon juice. Mix well and bring to a light boil. Cover and simmer for 45 minutes.

3. Best served as a side dish to accompany chicken or alongside white basmati rice or cauliflower rice.

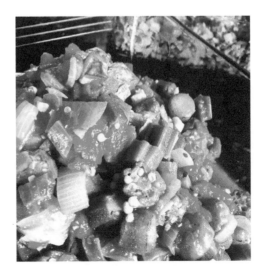

CHICKPEA & POTATO CURRY

This vegetarian dish is satisfying and super-healthy as a main or side dish. It can be doubled so you can enjoy it for couple of days and even take it with you for lunch. To up the protein and add a richer taste, you can add 1 lb. of cubed beef or chicken after you add the onions; cook everything for an extra 30 minutes and you will have a very nourishing meal.

HERE IS WHAT YOU NEED:

2 tablespoons coconut or olive oil

1 onion, chopped

1 yellow squash, diced

2 cups mini potatoes cut in half (or diced regular potatoes)

1 can organic chickpeas, drained (or 1 ½ cups cooked chickpeas)

1 cup water

2 teaspoons curry powder

1 teaspoon garam masala

1 teaspoon cumin

Salt and pepper

¼ teaspoon cinnamon (optional)

LET'S DO THIS:

1. In a heavy stove-to-oven skillet or pot (with a lid) heat the oil and sauté the onions lightly. Add the rest of the ingredients (except the water and spices), with breaks in between to allow for proper cooking. Let all ingredients cook for 5 more minutes.

2. Add the water and the seasonings (optional to add cinnamon). Mix together with a wooden spoon to spread the seasonings evenly. Bring to a gentle boil, lower the heat and cover. Let simmer for a few minutes.

3. Transfer to a 350°F oven for 30 minutes. When the potatoes are soft, the dish is ready to be served.

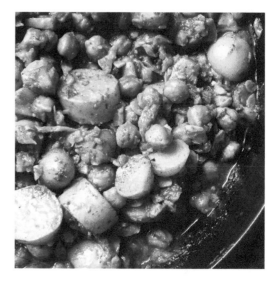

ROASTED CHERRY TOMATOES

You can use this delicious and fragrant recipe in so many ways: it can be a topping for pasta or rice, served as a side dish with a BBQ or grilled meat, or spread on a slice of toast like a bruschetta.

HERE IS WHAT YOU NEED:

1 lb. organic cherry tomatoes

¼ cup olive oil

4 garlic cloves, crushed

5-6 stems fresh thyme
(a sprinkle of
dried or fresh thyme
or oregano)

Salt and pepper

LET'S DO THIS:

1. Combine everything together in a large bowl and toss well.

2. Transfer to a ceramic dish and roast at 425°F for a half hour or until the tomatoes begin to burst.

3. Remove from the oven and let cool a bit before serving.

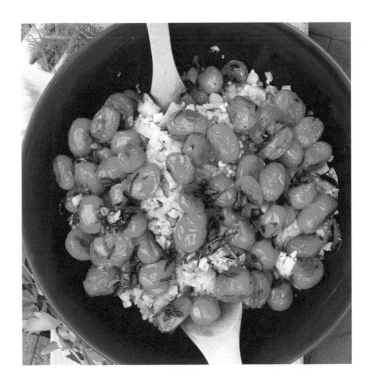

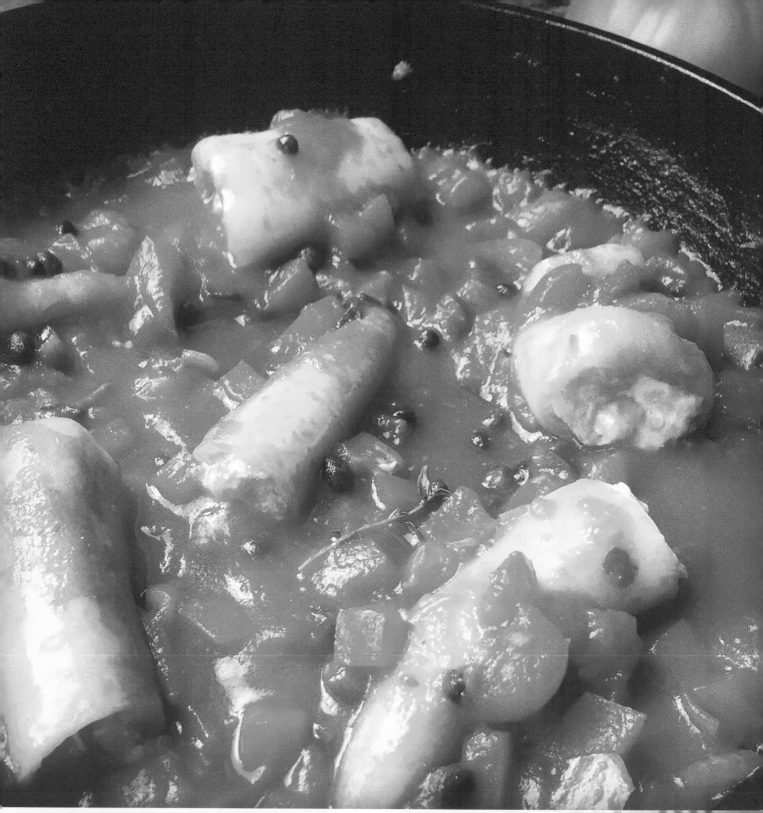

GOAT CHEESE STUFFED BANANA PEPPERS

Banana peppers are such a beautiful and delicate vegetable and often ignored because we don't really know what to do with them. Here is a simple recipe with wonderful flavors that can be a light dinner or an appetizer. I use organic goat cheese for the filling, but you can use any cheese you like.

HERE IS WHAT YOU NEED:

Sauce:

4 tablespoons coconut
  or olive oil

1 onion, chopped

1 shallot, chopped

1 large red tomato, diced

1 jalapeno pepper, diced tiny

1 tablespoon tomato paste

4 garlic cloves, minced

1 cup water

2 teaspoon dried oregano

Dash of chili pepper

Salt and pepper

Peppers:

3-5 banana peppers, cut in
  half horizontally

4 oz. organic goat cheese

3 tablespoons capers, rinsed

LET'S DO THIS:

1. In a large skillet, heat the oil and start sautéing all of the ingredients, adding them in the order listed, with breaks in between to allow each ingredient to sauté thoroughly. Finally, add the seasonings, and give the sauce a gentle swirl with a wooden spoon. Simmer for 5 minutes.

2. While the sauce is cooking, clean and cut the peppers and fill them with the cheese. Gently place them in the tomato sauce, sprinkle on the capers and cover with a lid. Let simmer for about 20 minutes. About mid-way, turn the peppers over once, and simmer for another 15 minutes.

CABBAGE STEAKS

This fun and easy side dish can accompany any meal or be the main dish. It is simple and different way to cook cabbage.

HERE IS WHAT YOU NEED:

1 head cabbage

Dried oregano

Garlic powder

Paprika

Red chili pepper flakes

Salt and pepper

2-3 tablespoons olive oil

LET'S DO THIS:

1. Cut the cabbage into steaks about ½-¾ " thick. Lay them flat on a cookie sheet lined with parchment paper. Brush with olive oil and sprinkle on the other seasonings.

2. Roast at 425°F for 30 minutes or until the tips of the leaves are golden brown.

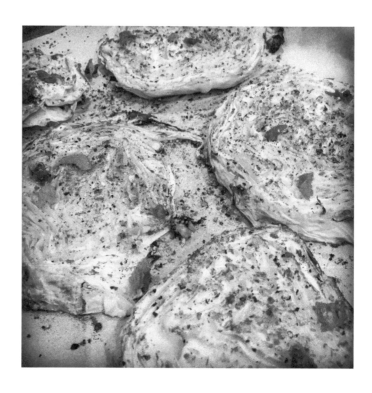

ROASTED RAINBOW POTATOES

This is a twist on a classic dish everyone loves. Next time you are grocery shopping, buy an array of colored potatoes: red, yellow, orange, purple and blue. You can also add a couple of beets for extra color and flavor as they take the same time to cook as potatoes. The mix of colors is beautiful and makes a great presentation. Have fun with it!

HERE IS WHAT YOU NEED:

6-7 large potatoes,
    or 10 small-medium ones
    (assorted colors)

¼ cup olive oil

Dried rosemary, pinch

Dried thyme, pinch

Salt and pepper

LET'S DO THIS:

1. Wash, dry and cut the potatoes into about 1"x1" pieces. Make sure they are dry.

2. Toss them in olive oil and transfer to a cookie sheet lined with parchment paper or a large ceramic dish. Sprinkle dried rosemary, sea salt, and pepper.

3. Roast at 425°F for 45 minutes or until the potatoes turn golden brown.

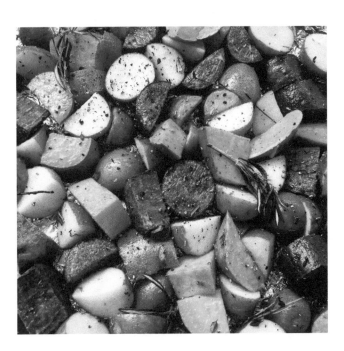

ROASTED EGGPLANTS WITH TAHINI

—

Eggplants are very popular in Israel and commonly found on restaurant menus. The combined taste of eggplant and tahini is fantastic, and this picturesque dish is sure to please all your guests.

HERE IS WHAT YOU NEED:

3 medium eggplants cut in half lengthwise (stem on)

3 tablespoons olive oil

Salt and pepper

Roasted tomatoes:

2 cups cherry tomatoes, halved

3 tablespoons olive oil

Salt and pepper

2 garlic cloves, minced

½ teaspoon dried thyme

½ teaspoon dried oregano

fresh thyme

Tahini dressing:

½ cup raw tahini

½ cup water

1 lemon, juice only

2 garlic cloves, minced

Salt and pepper

LET'S DO THIS:

1. Lay the eggplants on a flat baking dish lined with parchment paper skin side down. With a small sharp knife score X marks in the eggplant, being careful not to poke through the skin. Drizzle with olive oil and roast at 425°F for about 30-40 minutes until the eggplant starts to turn golden brown.

2. While the eggplants are roasting, toss the tomatoes with the seasonings and place in a small baking dish in the oven. At this point, you can add 2 sprigs of thyme on top for extra fragrance. If space does not allow the two vegetables to roast side by side, the eggplants and tomatoes can be on two different shelves in the same oven. Roast the tomatoes on 425°F for 20-30 minutes or until their juice bubbles out.

3. While the eggplants and the tomatoes are roasting, prepare the tahini dressing in a small bowl, combining all the ingredients and mixing them well.

4. To put it all together, let the eggplants cool a bit, then drizzle on the tahini sauce and top with the roasted tomatoes. Sprinkle a pinch of salt, black pepper and 1 tablespoon of olive oil just before serving.

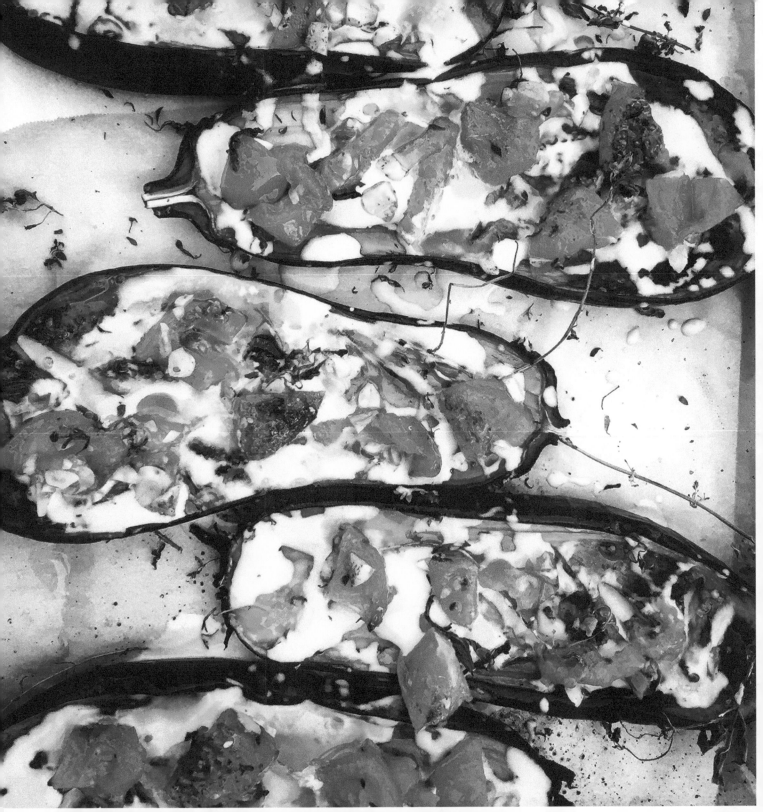

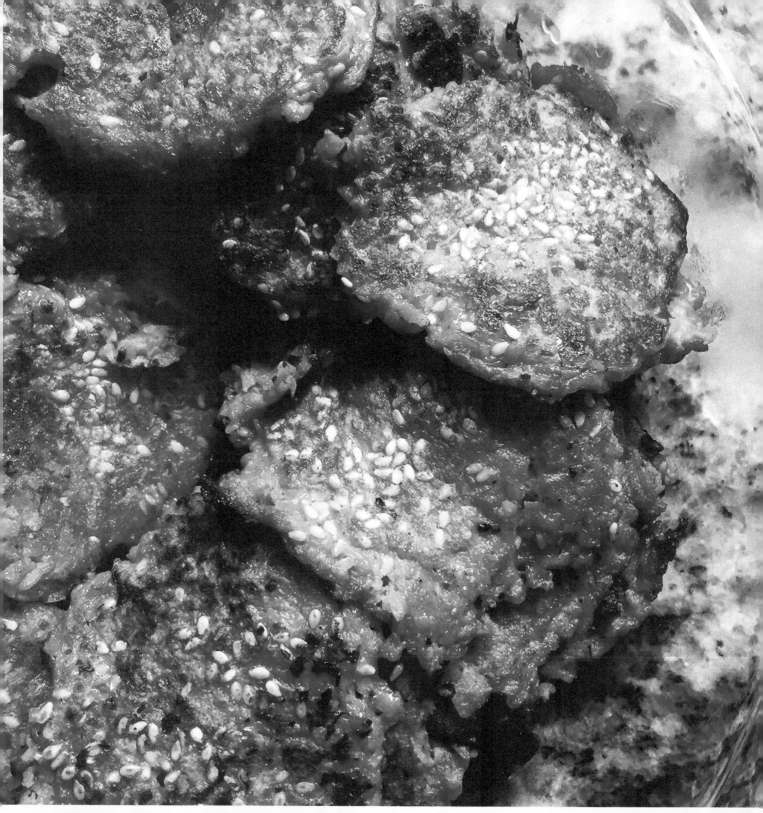

SWEET POTATO LATKES

Sweet potatoes are delicious and nutritious! While latkes are traditionally eaten for Chanukah, you may decide to enjoy these any time. Trust me, there won't be any leftovers, and if there are, you will have no complaints when you pack them in a lunch or have them the next day for breakfast!

HERE IS WHAT YOU NEED:

2-3 sweet potatoes, peeled and cut to about 1"x1" chunks

1 onion, cut into quarters

¼ cup arrowroot flour

½ cup almond meal

3 eggs

¼ teaspoon baking soda

Salt and pepper

¼ cup coconut or olive oil for frying

LET'S DO THIS:

1. Combine all the ingredients (except for the oil) in a food processor and process until a coarse but even mixture forms.

2. Heat a skillet with coconut oil on medium heat. Drop spoonful of the mixture, the size of small pancakes, and fry until the edges lighten.

3. Optional: sprinkle sesame seeds on top, then gently flip the latkes over.

4. When the latkes are ready, place them in a dish lined with paper towel, to absorb any extra oil. Serve warm.

CAULIFLOWER RATATOUILLE

Cauliflower is a very versatile vegetable, available all year round, and packed with lots of healthy nutrients. Since this vegetable has a bland flavor, you can dress it up or down and create an array of wonderful dishes. This recipe features stewed cauliflower florets in a rich and flavorful tomato sauce studded with black olives.

HERE IS WHAT YOU NEED:

1 cauliflower head, separated into florets

20 Kalamata olives, pitted

Parsley for garnish

Sauce:

4-5 tablespoon coconut or olive oil

1 large onion, diced

2 garlic cloves, minced

2 cups sweet peppers, any color, sliced into wedges

1 jalapeño pepper, diced to tiny pieces

1 14.5-oz can of organic tomato puree

2 tablespoons organic tomato paste

1 cup water

1 teaspoon paprika

1 teaspoon cumin

2 teaspoon dried oregano

¼ teaspoon cayenne pepper

Salt and pepper

LET'S DO THIS:

1. Add the oil to a large skillet on the stove on medium heat. Add sauce ingredients in the order they are listed and stir in between additions to make sure they are sautéed. Bring to a gentle boil and let it simmer covered for 5 minutes on low heat.

2. Uncover and gently place the cauliflower florets in the sauce.

3. Add the olives, distributing them evenly. Cover and simmer for another 20-30 minutes on low heat. Sprinkle with parsley (optional) and serve.

4. This dish will last in the fridge for a few days and can be a great companion to any chicken or fish dishes. It is also great by itself over basmati rice or quinoa, for a full, satisfying and nutritious dinner.

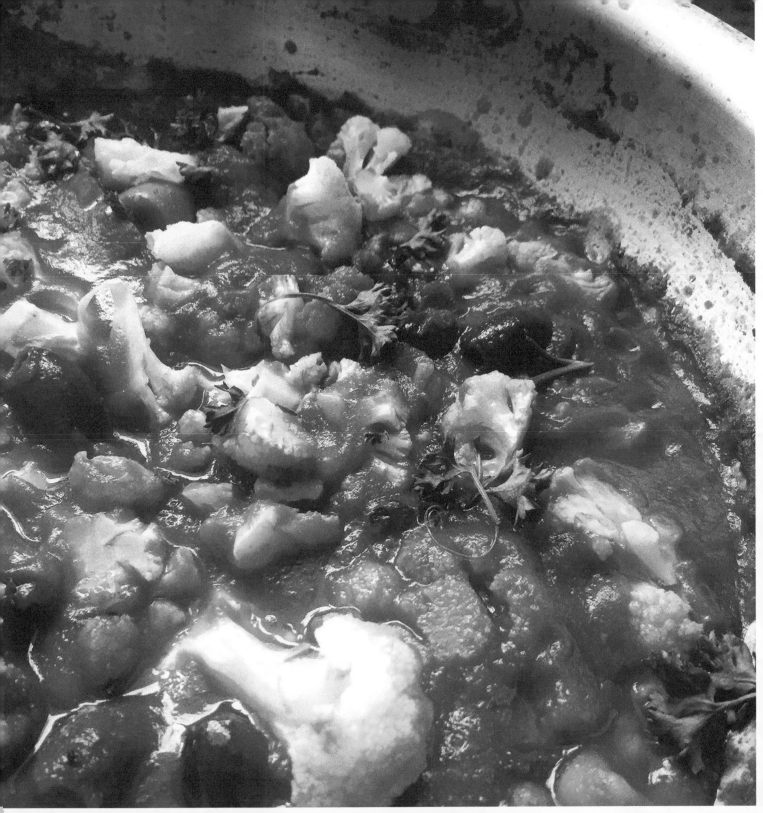

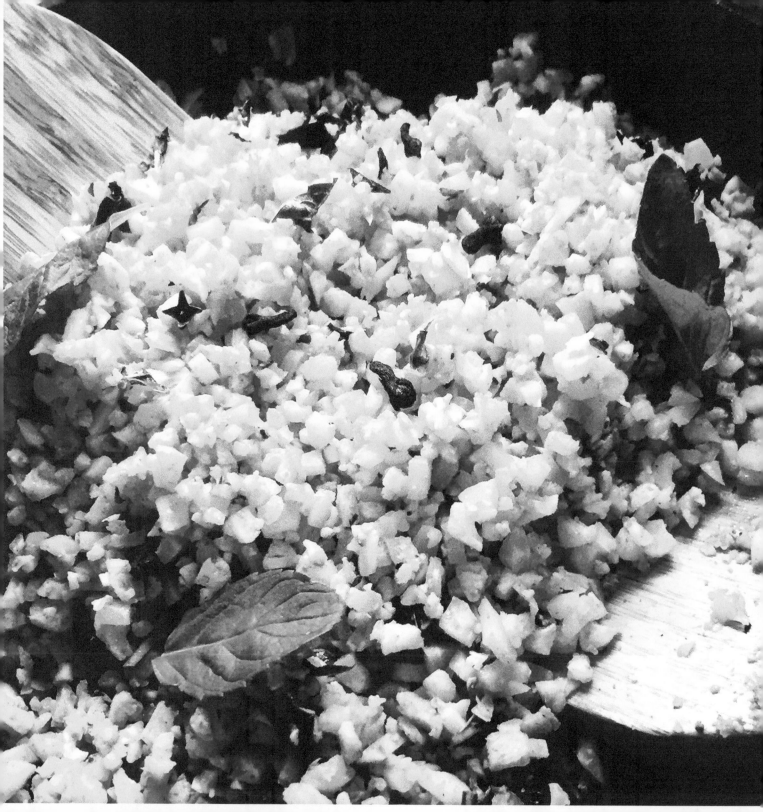

YELLOW CAULIFLOWER RICE

Cauliflower rice gained raves recently as a nutritious and convenient substitute for real rice. Here is a fun way to turn a bland dish to a vibrant and delicious side dish with extra antioxidants properties from the turmeric spice. It takes just a few minutes to prepare which is a huge plus in my book! Luckily, many grocery stores stock pre-shredded cauliflower, which cuts the preparation time by half. Leftovers are great reheated or served over a pile of greens with lemon juice as a salad the next day.

HERE IS WHAT YOU NEED:

1 head of cauliflower (or 1 bag pre-shredded cauliflower)

3 tablespoons coconut or olive oil

1 teaspoons turmeric

4-5 whole cloves

1 teaspoon sea salt

Freshly ground pepper

LET'S DO THIS:

1. Shred the cauliflower in a food processor until the pieces resemble grains of rice. Alternatively, use a bag of pre-shredded cauliflower.

2. Heat the oil in a wide skillet on the stove and add the cauliflower. Let sear for a few seconds and stir.

3. Add the spices and stir again. Let cook for 5 minutes total while stirring a couple more times. The cauliflower cooks quickly, and you want it to cook evenly yet el dente.

HEARTY CABBAGE STEW

This is a light yet very satifying dish. Enjoy it as a dinner on a cold day, or as a side dish next to beef or chicken.

HERE IS WHAT YOU NEED:

1 onion, chopped

1 head cabbage, chopped

1 can (14.5 ounces) organic stewed tomatoes or sauce

Or

2 fresh tomatoes, chopped

4-5 garlic cloves, minced

2 lemons, juice only

Salt and pepper

LET'S DO THIS:

1. Start by sautéing the onions in a large skillet for 5 minutes.

2. Add the cabbage and sauté for another 5 minutes.

3. Add the rest of the ingredients and stir well to combine. Bring to a light boil. Cover and simmer for 45 minutes on low heat.

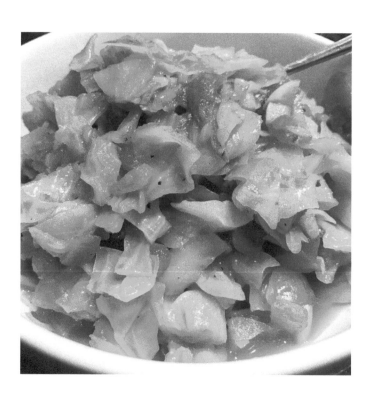

KOMBU, KALE & CHICKPEA SOUP

Don't let the word Kombu scare you...it is a kind of seaweed rich in iodine, calcium, and other essential minerals and contains enzymes that help to digest beans. This humble kelp can help reduce cholesterol and support thyroid functionality and more. You can find it in health food stores and some mainstream supermarkets (alongside other Asian foods). In this recipe, Kombu pairs with kale and beans to create a flavorful and healthy soup.

To get ready to make this recipe, you will have to soak the beans overnight. This easy step helps beans cook faster and makes them easier to digest. Simply place the beans in a bowl and fill it until the water is about 3" above the beans.

HERE IS WHAT YOU NEED:

Soup pot filled ¾ of the way with water

1 Kombu leaf

1½ cups mixed beans, such as lentils, chickpeas, and white beans (soaked in water overnight and rinsed before using)

2 tablespoons cumin

1 tablespoon sea salt

1 teaspoon apple cider vinegar

2 cups chopped kale

LET'S DO THIS:

1. Heat a pot of water until boiling. Add the beans / lentils, salt, cumin, vinegar, and Kombu.

2. Boil uncovered for 2 minutes. Cover and simmer for one hour on low heat.

3. Add the kale and simmer for 15 minutes. Remove the Kombu, chop it, and return it to the soup.

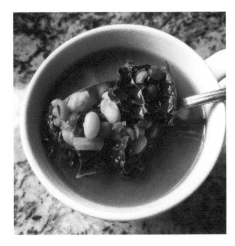

SPAGHETTI SQUASH WITH MUSHROOM RED SAUCE

With just a few simple ingredients, you can create a true gourmet dish! You can substitute the mushrooms for a pound of ground beef and make it a meal fit for carnivores. Either way will be delicious and I promise, everyone will love it!

HERE IS WHAT YOU NEED:

1 spaghetti squash

Parsley or cilantro (for garnish)

Sauce:

2 tablespoons olive oil

1 onion, chopped small

4 oz. mushrooms, chopped tiny

1 (14-ounce) can organic tomato sauce

1 (14-ounce) can organic diced tomatoes

2 garlic cloves, minced

1 teaspoon dried oregano

¼ teaspoon garlic powder

chili pepper powder, pinch

dried thyme, pinch

Salt and pepper

LET'S DO THIS:

1. Wash and dry the squash. Poke a few holes in its skin with a sharp knife. Either microwave on high for 10 minutes, or bake at 375°F for a half hour. Let cool and half the squash from tip to end. Remove all of the seeds.

2. Drizzle 1-tablespoon olive oil on each half, sprinkle with salt, and place the halves skin side up on a baking dish, with a crushed clove of garlic under each half. Bake at 375°F for 45 minutes. Take out and let cool a bit. Turn the squash skin side down, and fluff it with a fork to separate the flesh and emphasize its spaghetti-like strands.

3. While the squash is baking, prepare the sauce. In a large skillet, heat the oil and sauté the onions and the mushrooms. Add the tomato sauce, canned tomatoes, and seasonings. Mix well and let simmer for a half hour. Taste and adjust with salt and pepper if necessary.

4. Scoop the sauce over the squash and garnish with parsley or cilantro.

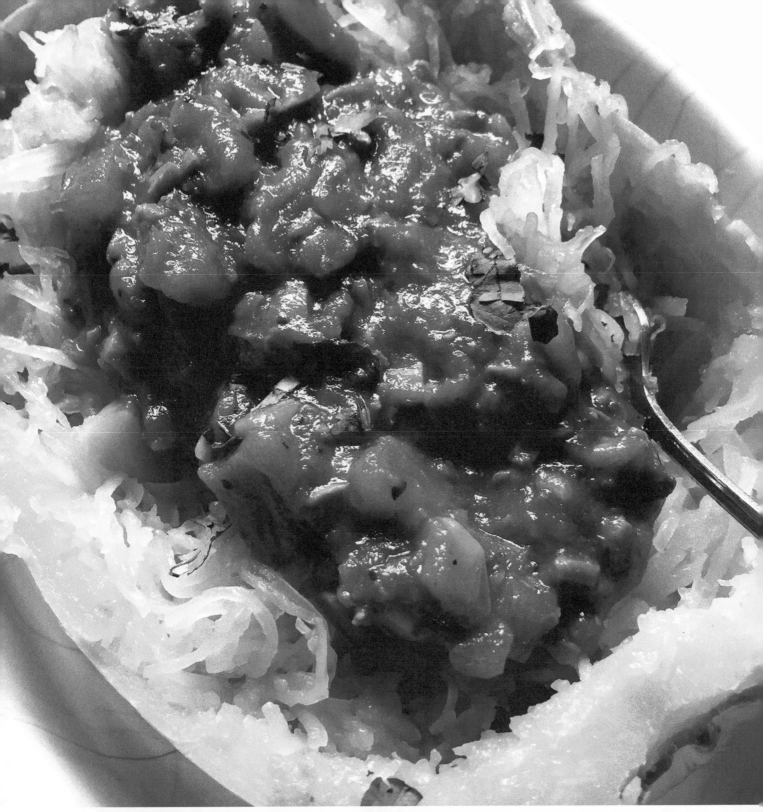

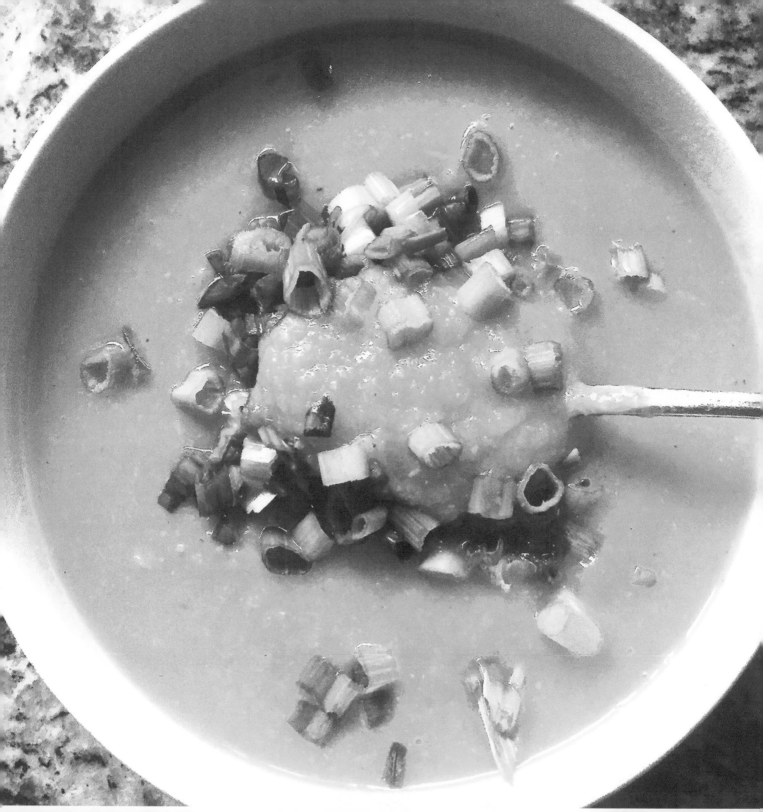

FALL FOR FALL SOUP

As soon as the temperatures outside begins to drop and the fall winds start picking up, my soup pot comes out of the cabinet and onto the stove! Soup is comforting, filling, and a great start to a meal. This soup will last for a few days in the fridge; you can pack it for lunch or serve it as a fast and healthy snack after school or work.

HERE IS WHAT YOU NEED:

¼ cup coconut or olive oil

Clean and cut the following to big chunks:

2 onions

5 carrots

2 cups Butternut squash

3 celery stalks

3 apples

2 yellow squash

4 garlic cloves

2 small sweet potatoes

2 (15-ounce) cans organic pumpkin

Seasoning:

1 tablespoon salt

1 teaspoon ginger powder

3" peeled fresh ginger, grated

¼ teaspoon cinnamon

1 teaspoon garlic powder

¼ cup maple syrup

Freshly ground pepper

LET'S DO THIS:

1. Heat the oil in a large soup pot and sauté the onions. Add the rest of the vegetables and apples, except for the canned pumpkin and continue to sauté on medium heat for 10 minutes.

2. Fill the pot ¾ full with water and add the seasonings and the canned pumpkin. Bring to a boil. Drop the heat to low and cover the pot. Simmer for one hour. Turn off the heat.

3. Using a handheld blender, process everything in the pot until smooth.

4. Optional: Garnish each soup bowl with chopped herbs, quinoa, scallions, rice, or croutons.

Seeds for Thought... To make a clean version of coconut milk, suitable for drinking or add to smoothies, simply blend 1 can coconut milk (organic and BPA free) with 4 cups of water. It is that easy!

I LIVE IN MY KITCHEN

ZUCCHINI BOATS

This is just a fun way to turn simple vegetables into a pretty and flavorful dish.

HERE IS WHAT YOU NEED:

3 zucchinis, cut in half lengthwise, cored (save the white part of the zucchini)

2 tablespoons olive oil

1 onion, chopped small

1 medium tomato, diced small

3 cups of mushrooms, chopped small

2 carrots, grated

2 garlic cloves, minced

1 egg, scrambled

½ teaspoon dried oregano

Salt and pepper

LET'S DO THIS:

1. Place the zucchini boats skin side down in a baking dish and sprinkle with salt and pepper.

2. Prepare the filling by sautéing the onions, tomatoes, mushrooms, carrots, white part of the zucchini, and garlic. Add the seasonings and cook for about 10 more minutes on medium-low heat until everything is incorporated and the mixture has thickened slightly. Remove the skillet from the stove, let the filling cool for 10 minutes, then add the egg and mix well.

3. Stuff the zucchini boats with the filling, using a spoon, and bake at 350°F for 30-45 minutes or until the filling starts to brown.

4. Optional: sprinkle full-fat organic mozzarella cheese on top and bake for another 10 minutes.

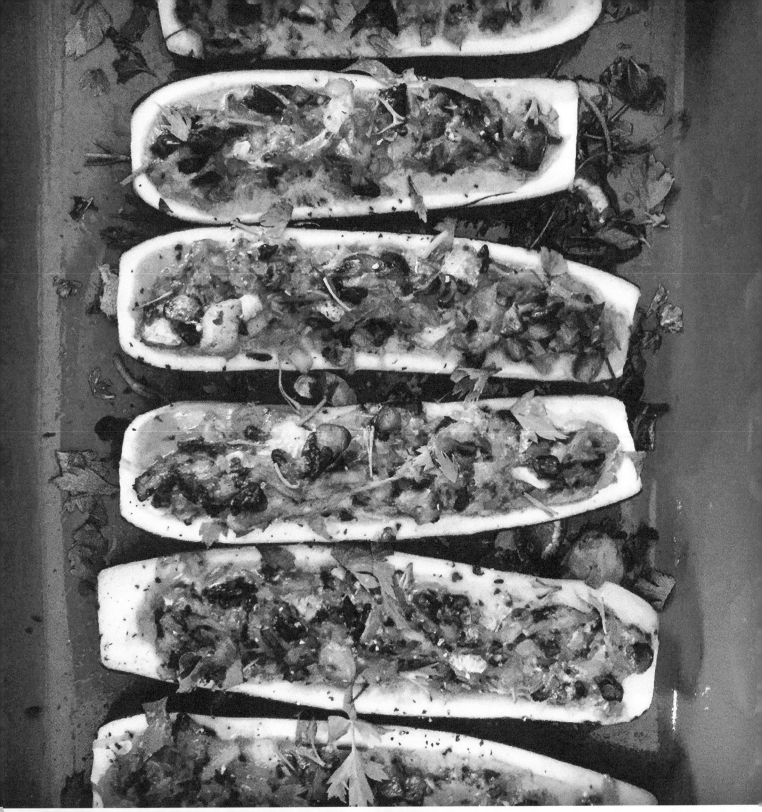

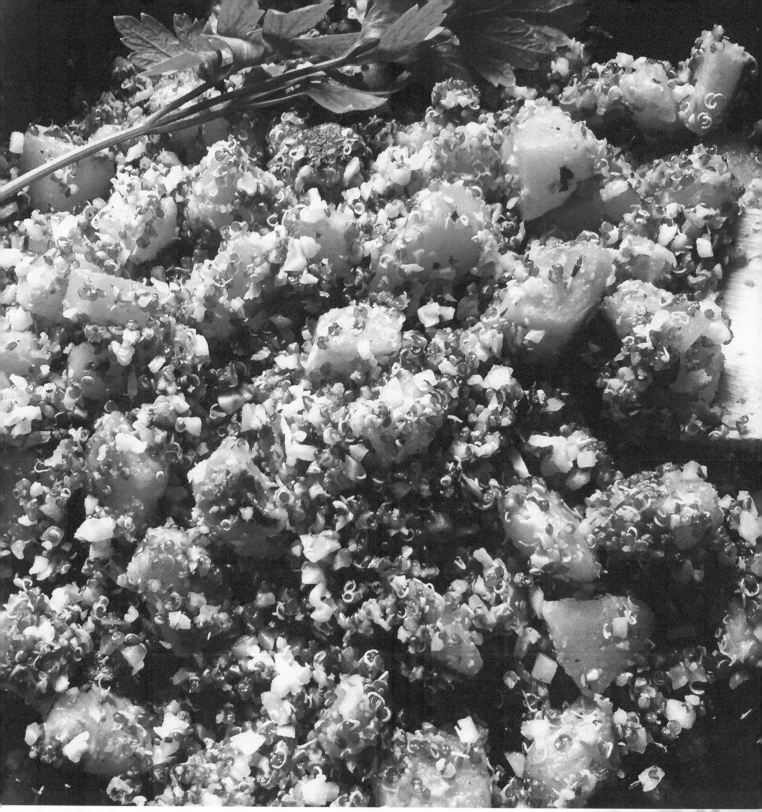

QUINOA & BUTTERNUT SQUASH MISHMASH

This satisfying dish is packed with an array of nutrients. It is a great dish to leave in the fridge and enjoy for a few days as a dinner, side dish, or packed lunch. But best of all, it is so easy to put together!

HERE IS WHAT YOU NEED:

3 tablespoons coconut or olive oil

1 lb. butternut squash, peeled and cubed

½ teaspoon sea salt

1 cup cooked red quinoa

2 cups shredded cauliflower

2 tablespoons coconut or olive oil

Pinch cinnamon

½ teaspoon cumin

½ lemon, juice only

Salt and pepper

LET'S DO THIS:

1. Sauté the butternut squash on medium-low heat in a large skillet with oil until soft, about 20-25 minutes. You can cover the skillet for 10 minutes to shorten the cooking time.

2. In the meantime, using a separate skillet, sauté the shredded cauliflower for 10 minutes. Add the cooked quinoa and seasonings and mix well.

3. Combine the cauliflower, quinoa and squash together in a larger bowl, sprinkle another pinch of salt, and serve.

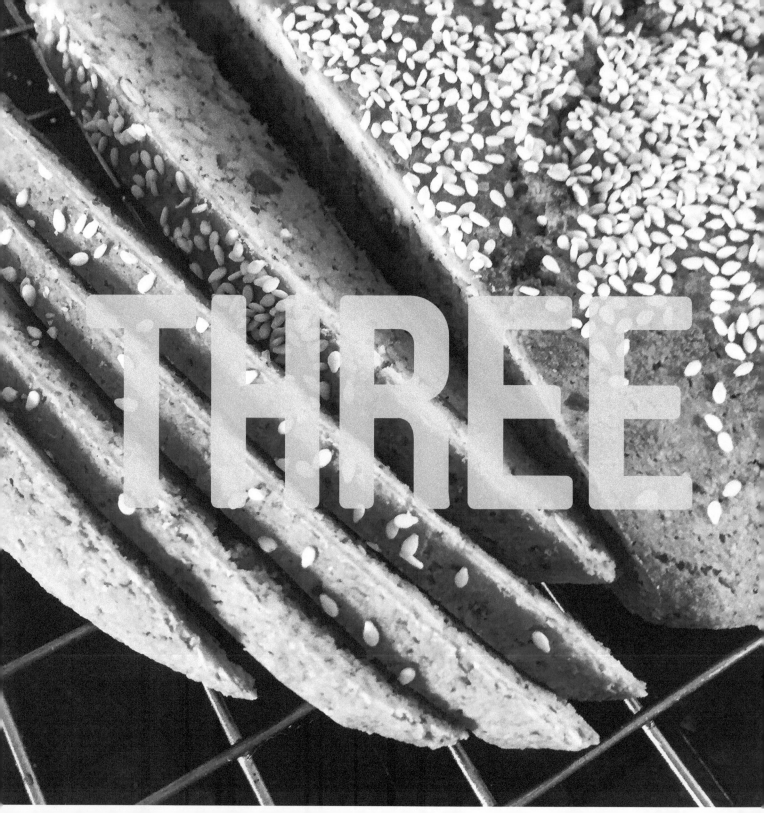

PIZZA & BREADS
Passion!

This section is for all the pizza and bread lovers out there! The recipes in this section are simple to prepare, but best of all, they are made with wholesome ingredients so you can enjoy your two favorite foods without the guilt.

PASSION FOR PIZZA

Who doesn't love pizza? After all, it is one of the most popular foods among kids and adults as one. There are many ways to make pizza healthier, starting with the crust. Here are two of my favorite crust recipes, one made from almond flour and the other made out of steamed cauliflower. You can also buy frozen, ready-made organic crust, to which you can add any homemade topping you like. Any of these options is preferable to the conventional version of pizza. And best of all, when you make it at home, you can enjoy pizza guilt-free!

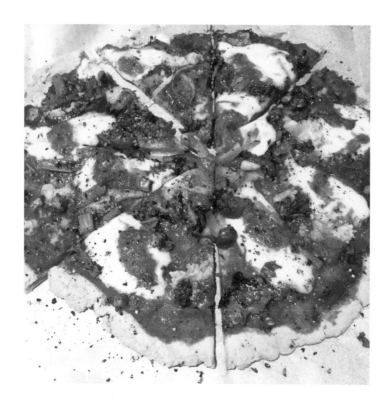

ALMOND MEAL CRUST

HERE IS WHAT YOU NEED:

1½ cups almond flour

1 tablespoon olive oil

1 teaspoon dried oregano

1 egg

¼ teaspoon baking soda

LET'S DO THIS:

1. Line a cookie sheet with parchment paper.

2. Combine all of the ingredients in a bowl and mix well. Use your hands if needed; it makes the process easier.

3. Place the dough in the middle of the pan and work with your hands to form a round crust ¼" thick.

4. Bake at 350°F for 10 min. Take it out and spread your favorite pizza toppings on the crust.

5. Bake for another 15 minute or until the edges of the crust become golden.

CAULIFLOWER CRUST

HERE IS WHAT YOU NEED:

2 ½ cups shredded cauliflower

2 eggs

¼ cup coconut flour (or other flour)

1 tablespoon olive oil

1 teaspoon garlic powder

1 teaspoon dried oregano

Salt and pepper

LET'S DO THIS:

1. Boil the shredded cauliflower until soft, about 10 minutes, and drain well trough a strainer. Use the back of your hands gently to force the access water to drain.

2. Combine the cauliflower and all the ingredients in a food processor until smooth and well-blended.

3. On a cookie sheet lined with parchment paper, shape the "dough" into a circle or rectangle, and flatten it with the heels of your hands until it is about ¼" thick.

4. Bake at 400°F for 15 minutes.

5. Remove from the oven, add your favorite topping, and bake until the edges of the crust turn golden brown (approximately 15 more minutes).

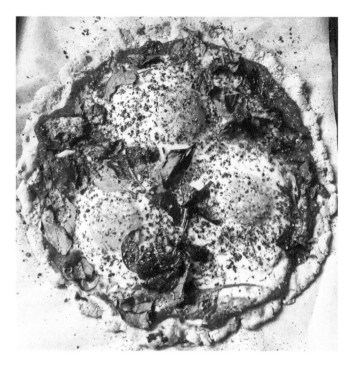

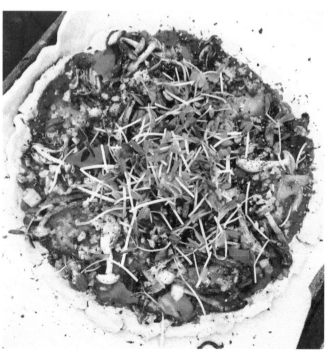

PIZZA TOPPINGS

The sky is the limit in terms of what can top a pizza. Here are some ideas for toppings, but you and your family can get creative and decorate each pizza as you see fit. Leftovers like roasted chicken and vegetables over red sauce are one of my favorite options for topping. The best accompaniment to a pizza is a large fresh green salad for a complete and nutritious meal.

EGG PIZZA:
Red sauce (pizza or marinara sauce), 3 whole eggs, dried oregano, fresh spinach leaves, and olive oil. Bake as instructed until the eggs are cooked.

WHITE PIZZA:
Prepare "white sauce" with 2 beaten eggs, crushed garlic, dried oregano, salt and pepper, and 1 tablespoon olive oil and mix well. Pour over the crust. Optional: sprinkle organic mozzarella cheese on top or sliced fresh tomatoes.

MUSHROOM PIZZA:
Red sauce topped with sautéed mushrooms and onions.

TOMATO AND BASIL PIZZA:
Red sauce, sliced fresh tomatoes, basil leaves, organic mozzarella discs, salt and pepper, dried oregano.

GOAT CHEESE PIZZA:
Red sauce, sliced fresh tomatoes, oregano, olive oil, goat cheese, spinach leaves.

ROASTED VEGETABLES PIZZA:
Red sauce, roasted vegetables like mushrooms, sweet potato, or cauliflower. Leftover dinner like chicken or vegetables makes great pizza topping.

OLIVES AND ARTICHOKE PIZZA:
Red or white sauce, halved artichoke hearts, halved cherry tomatoes, and oregano.

PESTO PIZZA:
Pesto sauce topped with any roasted vegetables and organic mozzarella cheese.

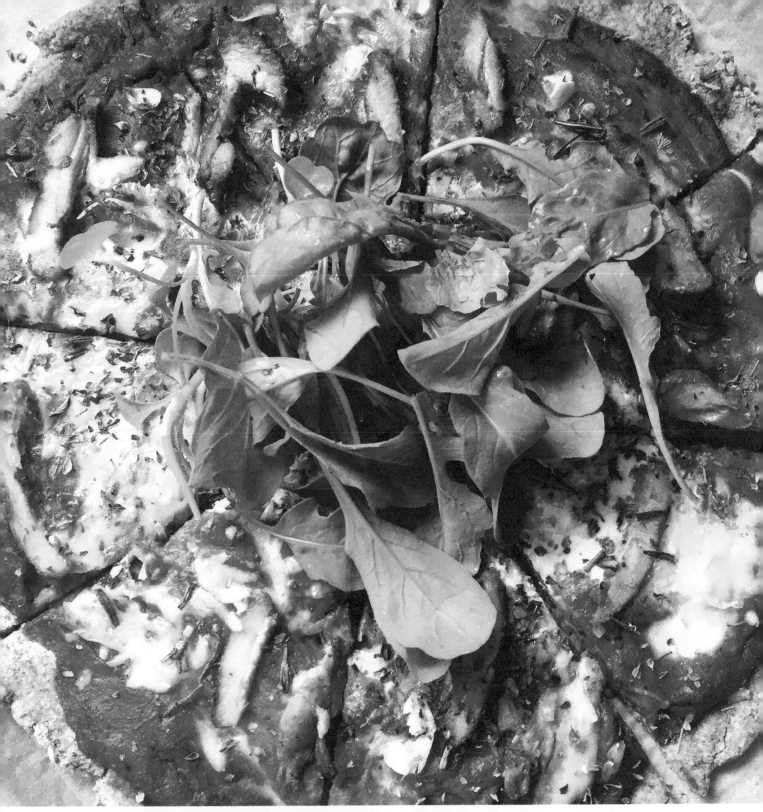

BETTER THAN BREAD

If you decided to avoid white flour and conventional baked goods, but you miss a piece of warm bread with butter, this recipe is for you. You can whip up this recipe in less than 5 minutes and enjoy a healthful piece of bread.

HERE IS WHAT YOU NEED:

2 ½ cups almond flour

½ cup arrowroot flour

½ cup raw pumpkin seeds

1 ½ teaspoon baking soda

2 pinches of sea salt

2 eggs

2 tablespoons honey

2 tablespoons apple cider vinegar

Sprinkle of sesame or caraway seeds as garnish (optional)

LET'S DO THIS:

1. Mix all the ingredients together in a large bowl using a mixer on low speed or by hand, with a large spoon.

2. Pour the dough into the middle of a pan lined with parchment paper and arrange it with your hand or a back of a wooden spoon into a round disc shape.

3. Sprinkle with either caraway seeds or sesame seeds, then score a large X across the top.

4. Bake at 350°F for 20 minutes until it turns light golden color.

Seeds for Thought... Organic Apple Cider Vinegar is known for its many health benefits and a good staple to have in the kitchen. Add it to soups and salad dressings for added zesty flavor. Some of its believed benefits include: reduce bloating, keeps you full longer, a source of probiotics, detoxifies, lower blood pressure, fights allergies and much more.

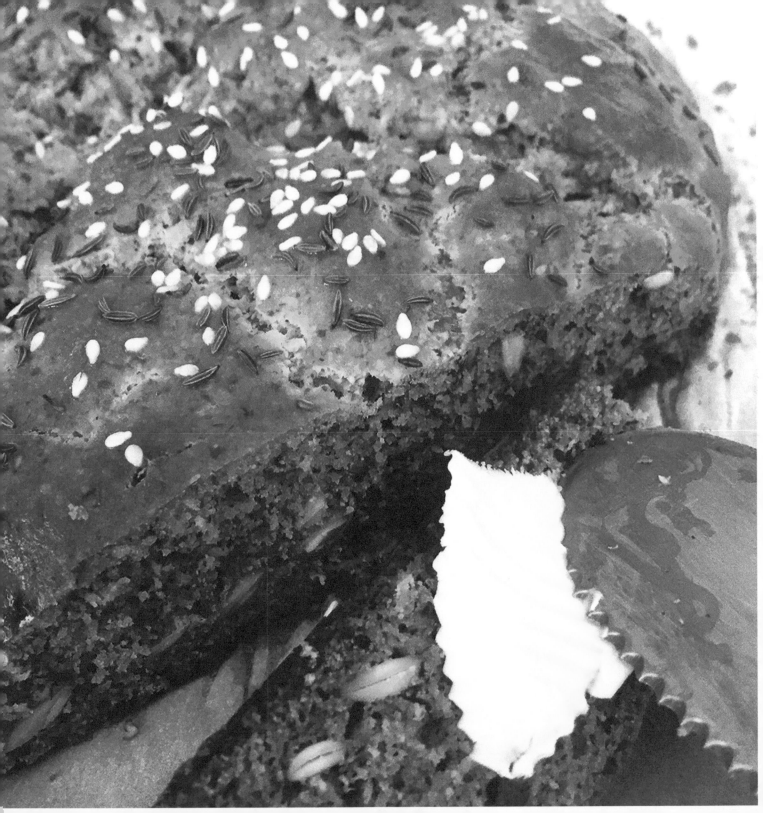

CARING CARROT MUFFINS

These carrot muffins are packed with wholesomeness and so easy to make. I like them plain or topped with a thin layer of butter for a satisfying and healthy snack. You can even top them with your favorite icing to please the guests with a sweet tooth.

HERE IS WHAT YOU NEED:

3 medium carrots

4 eggs

¼ cup coconut sugar

¼ cup melted coconut oil

⅓ cup dry quinoa

1 cup Einkorn flour
    (or spelt flour)

¼ teaspoon baking powder

Sprinkle of cinnamon

½ cup chopped pecans or
    chocolate chips (optional)

LET'S DO THIS:

1. Using a food processor on medium-low speed, start adding the ingredients in the order they appear in the recipe. If using chocolate chips, add them last, and mix gently.

2. Scoop into 12 cupcakes liners in a muffin pan. Garnish each with a few chocolate chips, and bake at 350°F for 25 minutes.

3. Let cool on a cooling rack.

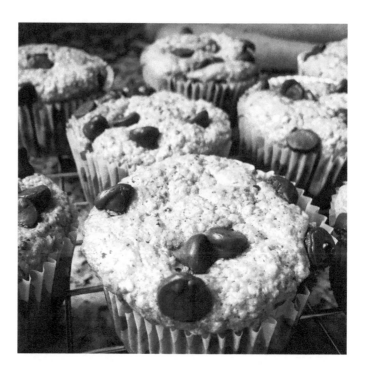

CARROT BREAD

This one goes out to all the bread lovers! The recipe uses a small bag of mini carrots, but you can also use regular carrots. This is savory bread, however, if you like your bread a bit sweeter, add ½ cup coconut sugar or 3 tablespoons maple syrup to the batter.

HERE IS WHAT YOU NEED:

2 eggs

1 bag mini carrots (12-oz)

2 tablespoons coconut sugar

2 tablespoons apple
cider vinegar

Pinch salt

1 cup almond meal

1 cup spelt flour

¼ cup flax seed meal

½ teaspoons baking soda

Sesame seeds for
garnish (optional)

LET'S DO THIS:

1. In a food processor, add the above ingredients in the order they appear and blend until they combine, pausing between each addition.

2. Pour the batter into a loaf pan lined with parchment paper and sprinkle sesame seeds on top.

3. Bake at 350°F for 30 minutes.

4. Let cool on a cooling rack.

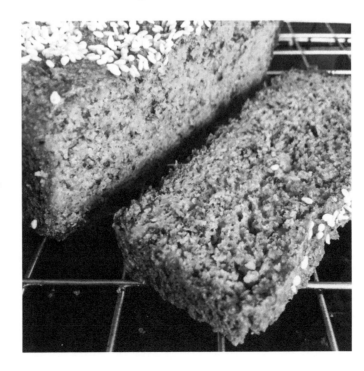

MY FAMOUS HEAVENLY BANANA BREAD

An oldie but oh-so-goodie becomes super-healthy in this revised version. The name might fool you since it is more like dessert than bread but one thing is for sure, it is delicious! Ripe, brown bananas are perfectly ok to use here but also just ripe yellow bananas are great. Don't let the long ingredient list scare you; most are from the staples list in the beginning of the book. Moreover, cleanup is straightforward, because you are using one tool—the food processor or a blender—to combine ingredients. As usual, add the ingredients as listed, with short pulses in between to ensure everything is blended.

HERE IS WHAT YOU NEED:

½ cup coconut oil, melted

¼ cup coconut sugar

3 eggs

3 bananas (frozen and defrosted or fresh)

1 tablespoon vanilla

2 cups almond meal

¼ cup flaxseed meal

¼ cup coconut flour

¼ cup arrowroot flour

½ teaspoon baking powder

½ teaspoon baking soda

Pinch of sea salt

Optional:

Splash cinnamon

½ cup chocolate chips

¼ cup chopped pecans

LET'S DO THIS:

1. Using a food processor or blender, start adding the ingredients in the order they appear. Stop blending after the vanilla.

2. Add the dry ingredients and then blend again until everything is combined. You might have to stop one more time and use a spatula to help incorporate the dry ingredients into the batter. You should have a thick batter.

3. At this point, you can add the optional cinnamon, chocolate chips or chopped pecans. Mix lightly with a spatula by hand.

4. Transfer to a loaf pan lined with parchment paper.

5. Bake at 350°F for 40-45 minutes. It is ready when you touch the center of the bread either with your fingers or a back of a spoon and it feels firm.

Variation: Use 1 cup almond meal and 1 cup of Einkorn flour instead of the other flours.

Seeds for Thought... Einkorn flour is made from ancient grains, minimally processed, and contains more nutrients and less gluten than regular white flour.

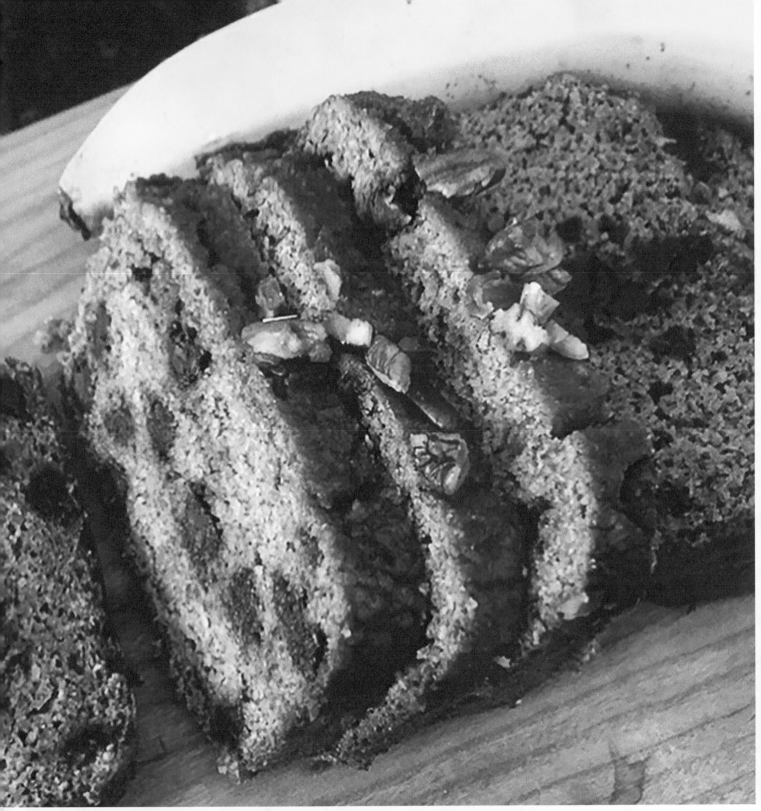

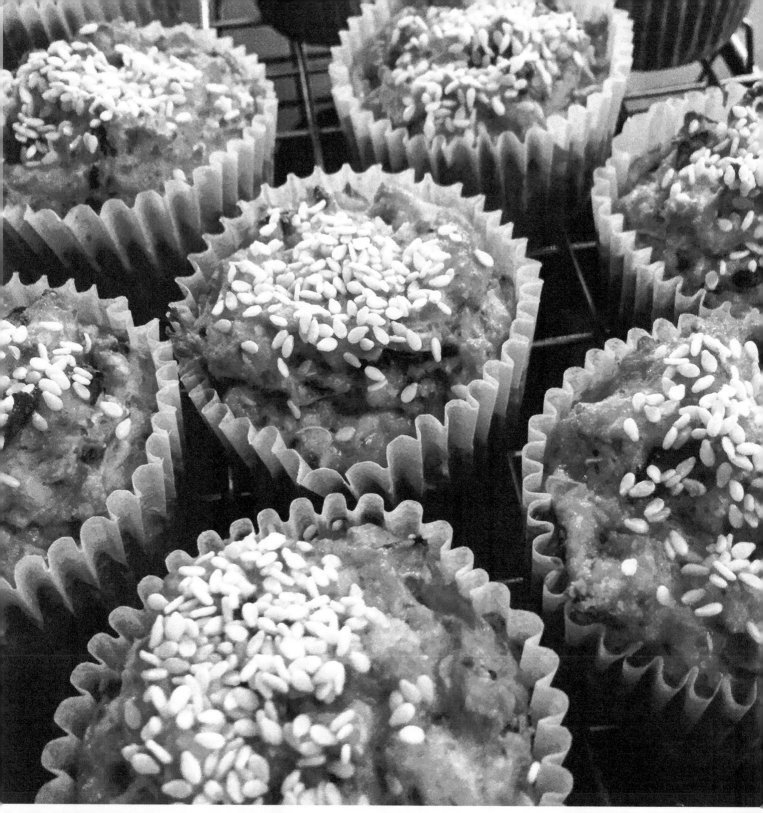

YELLOW SQUASH MUFFINS

This savory snack is reminiscent of zucchini bread, built into a muffin shape. These muffins are great to pack for lunch or as a healthy snack, with a dalope of strawberry jelly or almond butter on top.

HERE IS WHAT YOU NEED:

2 yellow squash, grated and squeezed through a strainer, to remove the liquid

4 eggs

¾ cup almond meal

¼ cup coconut flour

¼ cup flaxseed meal

¼ teaspoon baking soda

½ teaspoon garlic powder

Salt and pepper for taste

1 grated sweet potato (optional)

LET'S DO THIS:

1. Mix all the ingredients in a large bowl. If the batter seems too dry, add one more egg. Season with the garlic powder, sea salt and black pepper to taste.

2. Scoop the mixture into a parchment-lined muffin pan. Sprinkle sesame seeds on each muffin.

3. Bake at 350°F for 30 minutes, or until the tops of the muffins are golden.

4. Store in a Ziploc™ bag or container in the fridge.

5. Optional: You can bake the batter in a rectangular baking glass dish and serve this as a quiche. Bake as instructed and cut into squares for easy serving.

BREAKFAST-ALL-DAY MUFFINS

My family just loves eggs in any shape or form for breakfast, lunch or dinner. When in doubt and there is no dinner to be found, we eat eggs. Sunny side up or scrambled will do but always with a side of vegetables to make it a complete meal.

These muffins are super easy to make and everyone would love to pack them for lunch or breakfast on the run. If you cannot find Brussels sprouts, don't worry! You can substitute them with shredded carrots, onions, cauliflower or any combination of vegetables you like.

HERE IS WHAT YOU NEED:

8 eggs, scrambled

10 ounces shredded Brussels sprouts, about 2 heaping cups

½ teaspoon sea salt

¼ teaspoon black pepper

¼ cup water

¼ cup kefir (optional)

½ cup crumbled full-fat feta cheese for garnish before baking (optional)

LET'S DO THIS:

1. In a large bowl combine all of the ingredients and mix very well.

2. Line cupcakes pan with 12 parchment liners and fill them up almost to the top. Sprinkle with cheese before baking.

3. Bake at 350°F for 25-30 minutes or until you notice the edges of the muffins turn golden brown color. Let cool. Can be stored in the refrigerator for up to a week.

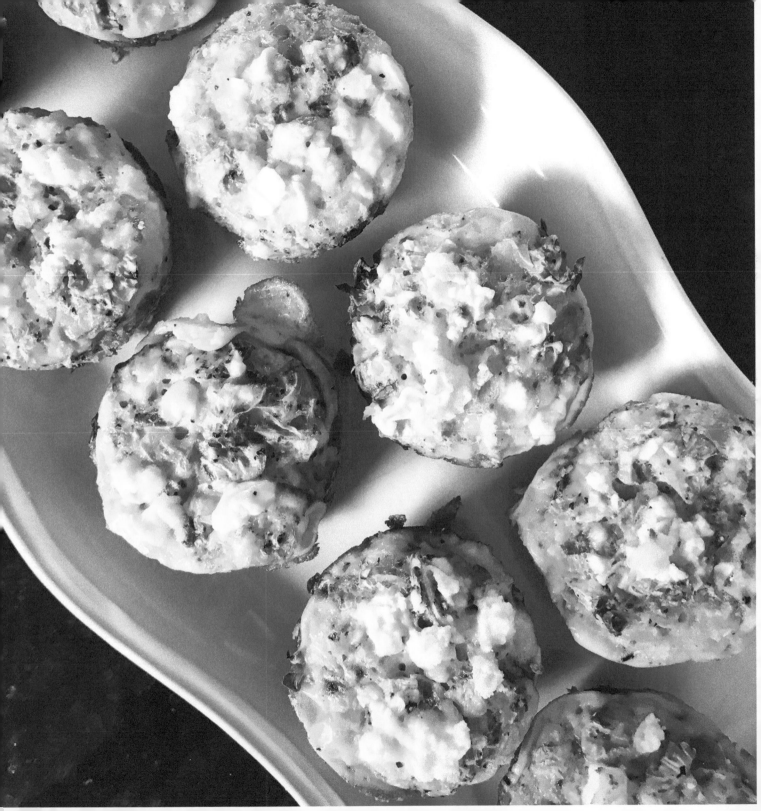

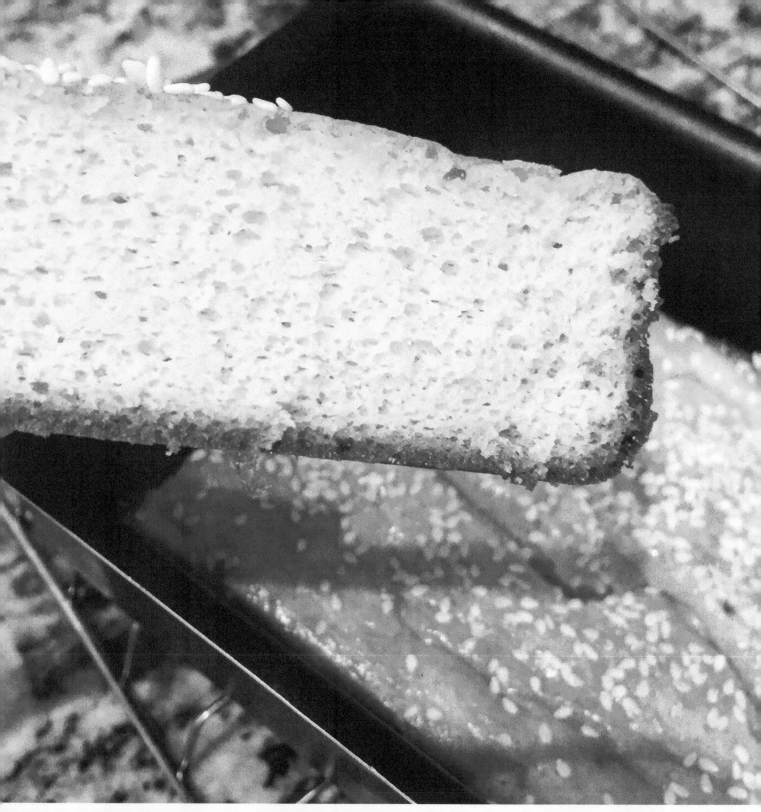

TAHINI BREAD

Tahini has been a staple in my home growing up, as it is a very common item in the Israeli cuisine. There are so many wonderful recipes using raw tahini, from savory sauces to sweet desserts. You can use it right out of the jar and drizzle over fish or a salad or add seasonings to create new flavors. It is rich in nutrients and healthy fats, and it is minimally processed. In this recipe we use tahini to make flourless bread. Enjoy a slice with fruit jam or butter on top as a snack or breakfast on the go.

HERE IS WHAT YOU NEED:

4 eggs

6 tablespoons raw tahini

2 tablespoons honey or maple syrup

1 teaspoon baking powder

Pinch of sea salt

Sesame seeds to sprinkle on top before baking

LET'S DO THIS:

Using a whisk, mix everything together until a smooth and loose batter forms. Pour into a lightly greased loaf pan, sprinkle with sesame seeds (optional) and bake at 350°F for 20-25 minutes or until it turns a golden color and the edges start to separate slightly from the pan.

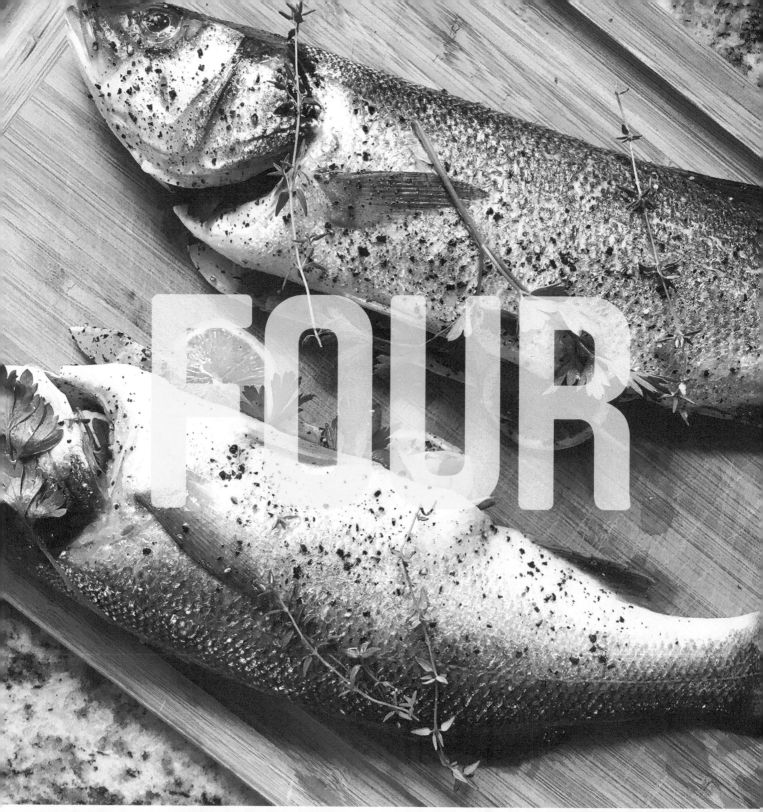

FISH
So Fresh!

Fish is a great option for a quick and healthy dinner. It takes only a few minutes to cook, is high in protein and omega-3 fatty acids, and can be easily dressed with any of your favorite spices.

SALMON WITH PARSLEY AIOLI

———

Salmon and other cold-water fish are an easy, quick, and substantial dinner options. They are excellent sources of Omega-3 fatty acids and other essential nutrients. For these reasons, I recommend you eat fish at least once or twice a week. This healthy and aromatic salmon dish uses a few simple ingredients to transform a familiar fish into an aromatic delight. The sesame seeds add crunch and a nutty flavor while the parsley aioli adds a garlic-infused twang.

HERE IS WHAT YOU NEED:

Salmon fillets (about 3-5 pieces)

1 tablespoon coconut or olive oil

1 tablespoon olive oil

Salt and pepper

1 tablespoon black and white sesame seeds (or just white sesame)

Parsley aioli:

¼ cup olive oil

1 cup parsley (or a bunch), chopped

2 garlic cloves, chopped

Juice from 1 lemon

Salt and pepper

LET'S DO THIS:

1. Combine all the ingredients for the parsley aioli in a tall jar and process with a hand-held blender until you have a smooth paste. (A small food processor can be used as well.)

2. Pat the salmon dry and coat lightly with a little olive oil. Sprinkle all over with sesame seeds, salt and pepper.

3. Warm a skillet with coconut oil and start searing the salmon, skin side up first, for about 4 minutes. Flip the fillet over when you see the edges of the fish turn a lighter color for another 3 minutes.

4. Transfer the salmon to a platter and scoop a spoonful of the parsley aioli onto each piece.

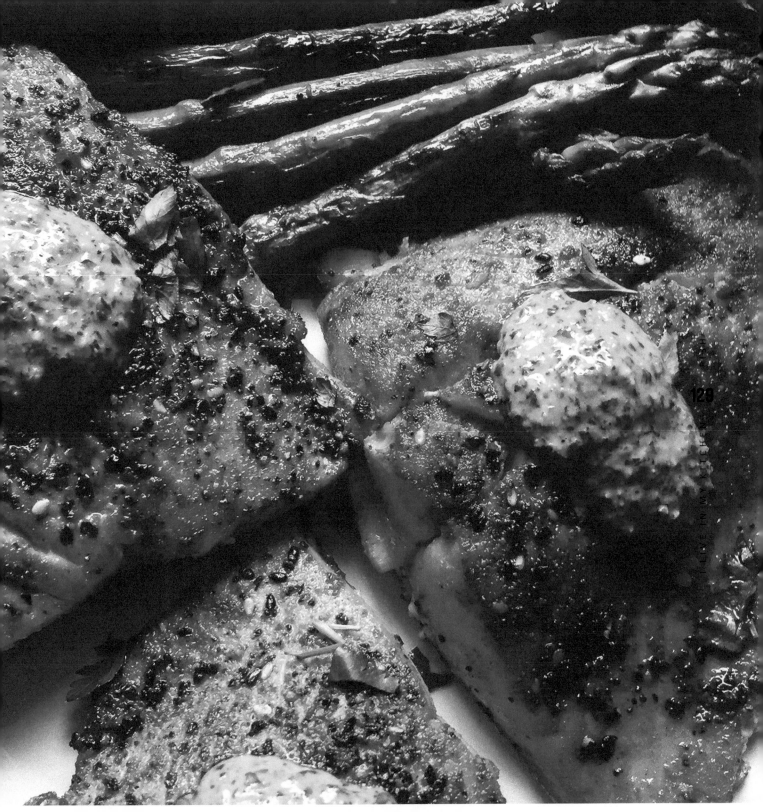

INDIAN-INSPIRED SALMON

Spices play a major role in my kitchen. Spices allow us to be creative and adventurous with our cooking and best of all, they turn any bland meal to an exciting culinary experience. This recipe uses Indian inspired seasonings to dress up a bland fish in just a few minutes.

HERE IS WHAT YOU NEED:

4 portions of salmon (or a whole fillet)

1-2 tablespoons olive oil

1 tablespoon coconut oil

Salt and pepper

Curry powder (¼ teaspoon or a sprinkle per portion)

Garlic powder (¼ teaspoon or a sprinkle per portion)

Black or white sesame seeds (sprinkle lightly)

LET'S DO THIS:

1. Lay the salmon, skin side down, on a large plate and pat dry. Drizzle with olive oil and spread it evenly with your hands. Sprinkle with salt and pepper, curry, and sesame seeds. You just want a thin layer of each of the spices. At this point, you can store the fish in a Ziploc® bag in the fridge for up to 24 hours or cook it right away.

2. In a large skillet, warm the coconut oil. Make sure the oil is hot enough for searing. Sear the salmon, skin side up first, for 3-4 minutes. Flip to the other side and sear for 5 more minutes. The cooking time depends on the thickness of the fish; generally speaking, thicker fillets take longer to cook. Use a sharp knife to make a small slit in the middle of the fish, to check if it is done..

Optional: Once you have flipped the salmon, add some peeled garlic cloves above and below the fish

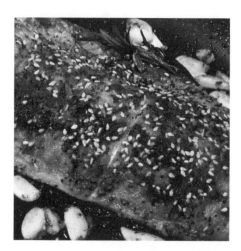

COD WITH CAPERS

The best recipes are the simplest ones! Here is a recipe that is light, fresh, and super-easy to make. This dinner will take 15 minutes to prepare—how can you beat that?

HERE IS WHAT YOU NEED:

1 lb. wild-caught cod (approximately)

4-5 tablespoons almond meal

2 tablespoons coconut oil

Sauce:

1-2 shallots, chopped

½ cup water

1 lemon, juice only

2 tablespoons capers, rinsed

Salt and pepper

LET'S DO THIS:

1. Clean and dry the fish. Place it on a cutting board and sprinkle with the almond meal. Season with salt and pepper.

2. In a large skillet, warm up the coconut oil. Sauté the fish until golden on each side, using low to medium heat, about 4-5 minutes each side. With a wide spatula, transfer the fish to a serving plate.

3. In the same skillet, sauté the shallots lightly. Add water, lemon juice, capers, salt and pepper. Scrape the bottom of the pan to get out all of the flavors. Let the sauce simmer for 3 minutes, until reduced by half. Pour over the fish just before serving.

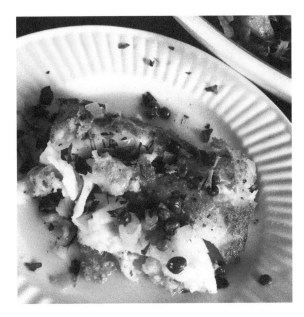

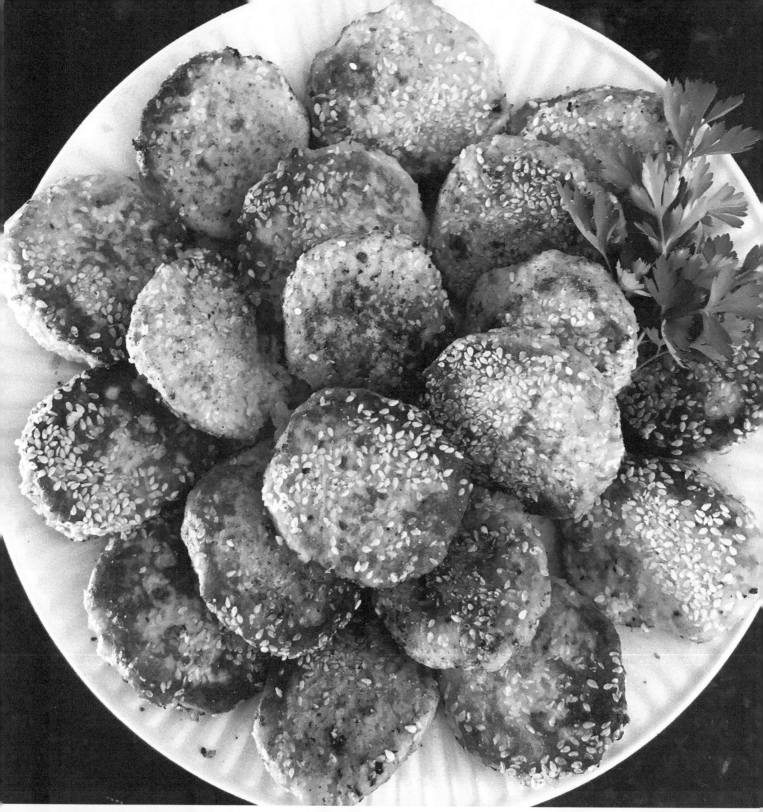

SALMON CUTLETS

If you are on the look for a new and exciting salmon recipe, you are for a treat! In this dish, the salmon changes its shape and becomes a cutlet; even kids will dare to try. This recipe is easy, delicious, and made out of super healthy ingredients.

HERE IS WHAT YOU NEED:

1 lb. salmon, skin off

1 onion, quartered

2 medium sweet potatoes peeled and cut into chunks

2 eggs, scrambled

½ teaspoon sea salt

¼ teaspoon garlic powder

¼ teaspoon dried thyme (optional)

Freshly ground pepper

¼ cup sesame seeds

2-4 tablespoons coconut oil for frying

LET'S DO THIS:

1. Place the potatoes and onions in a food processor and process until rice like consistency forms.

2. Place the mixture in a large stainer over a large bowl and press to extract the liquid out. Transfer mixture into a dry bowl.

3. Using the food processor again, no need to wash the container, process the salmon until coarsely chopped. Add the salmon to the potatoes and onion mixture.

4. Add the eggs and seasonings to the bowl. Mix well until an even consistency forms.

5. Warm up the oil in a skillet over medium-low heat. Using your hands, form cutlets and lightly fry them, about 4 minutes each side. Sprinkle sesame seeds on each cutlet once they are cooking on the first side. Turn to the other side only when you notice that the edges of the cutlets turn white and they feel firm enough to flip.

GINGER SALMON

A simple, beautiful dish. Just sprinkle the seasonings on the salmon fillets before searing, and finish the dish with more fresh ginger and lemon wedges. Serve on a bed of fresh greens sprinkled with shredded cauliflower or any other green side dish.

HERE IS WHAT YOU NEED:

4 salmon fillets

Seasoning to sprinkle
   over each fillet:

Pinch salt and pepper

Pinch chili powder

Pinch of dry ginger

1" fresh ginger, grated

Lemon wedges, for serving

LET'S DO THIS:

1. Spread all the seasoning on the fish and sauté in a heavy skillet for about 4 minutes on each side, starting with skin side up.

2. Serve with fresh ginger on top and a wedge of lemon.

3. Optional: instead of using the stove, you can bake at 425°F for 25 minutes.

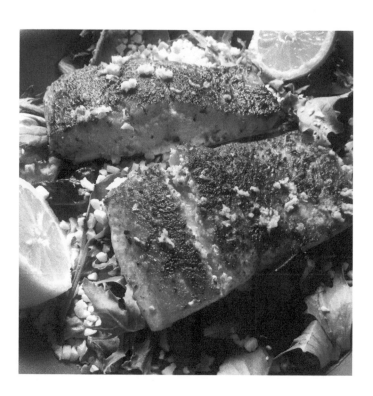

SALMON IN A POCKET

Once you try this recipe once, you won't have to look at the written recipe again because it is that simple to prepare. The salmon comes out moist and melts in your mouth due to the method of preparation. Even picky eaters would love this dish with a side of mashed potatoes or plain rice.

HERE IS WHAT YOU NEED:

Cut a large square of parchment paper or foil and lay it on a cookie sheet.

1 Salmon fillet, patted dry

2 tablespoons olive oil

2 sprigs of fresh thyme, rosemary, or oregano (or 1 teaspoon of dried herbs like thyme, rosemary, or oregano)

½ lemon, juice

3 garlic cloves, halved

Sea salt and pepper

LET'S DO THIS:

1. Drizzle 1 tablespoon of oil in the middle of the parchment paper or foil. Place the salmon fillet on top.

2. Sprinkle the rest of the seasonings all over the salmon.

3. Bring the two edges of the parchment paper or foil together and fold them tightly. Do the same with the other sides creating a 'pocket' for the fish.

4. Bake in the oven at 425°F for 20-25 minutes. Take out of the oven. Unfold the paper and serve with a drizzle of lemon juice.

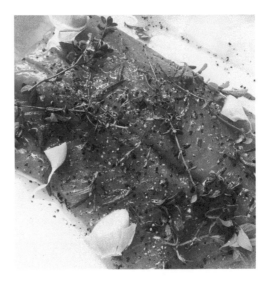

COD IN TAHINI SAUCE

———

Raw tahini is a great addition to a fish dish and typical in the Mediterranean cuisine. The creaminess of the tahini sauce complements perfectly any fish. It takes just a few minutes to prepare, and the result is a gourmet main dish everyone would love.

HERE IS WHAT YOU NEED:

2 tablespoons coconut oil

1-2 lbs. wild caught cod

1 red onion, quartered

3 garlic cloves, sliced

¼ cup raw tahini sauce

½ cup cherry tomatoes, halved

Salt and pepper

Fresh or dried thyme

1 lemon

LET'S DO THIS:

1. In a cast iron skillet sauté the onions in oil lightly.

2. Move the onions to the side of the skillet and add the fish. After turning the fish to its other side, sprinkle on top with tahini, garlic, salt, and pepper and cook over medium-low heat for 5 minutes.

3. Add the tomatoes and thyme to the dish and either continue to cook for 10 more minutes on the stove or transfer to 400°F oven for 5-6 minutes. Drizzle with lemon juice before serving.

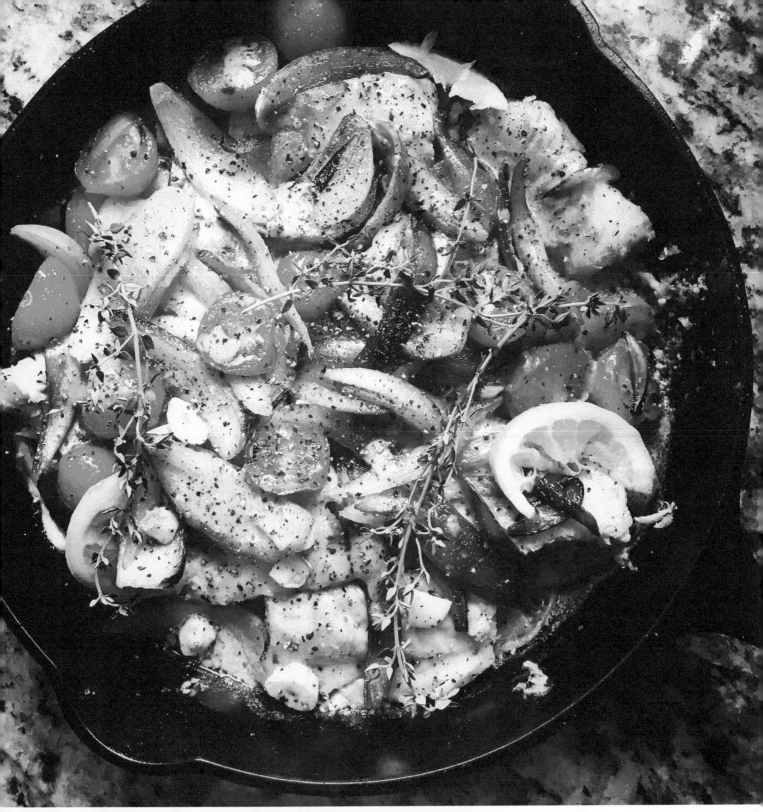

HADDOCK OVER LENTILS & KALE

This recipe is for a suggestion for a complete meal: fish, greens and lentils, but you can choose to make one dish or the other. Your choice! Both are simple and super-healthy choices.

HERE IS WHAT YOU NEED:

Greens and lentils:

1 cup sprouted lentils

3 cups water

2 tablespoons tomato paste

1 cup water

1 lemon, juice only

Salt and pepper

2 garlic cloves, minced

3 cups chopped kale

Fish:

1 tablespoon coconut oil

1 haddock fillet

1 tablespoon olive oil
(for spreading on the
fish before cooking)

1 teaspoon paprika

2 tablespoons sesame seeds

Salt and pepper

LET'S DO THIS:

Greens and lentils:

1. Cook lentils with water for 20 minutes, drain the water and place the lentils back in the pot.

2. Add all of the ingredients except the kale to the pot, Bring to a gentle boil. Lower the heat and cover. Simmer on low heat until the lentils reach a stew-like consistency about 20 minutes.

3. Add the kale and cook for 10 more minutes.

Fish:

1. Lay the fish on a cutting board and spread on a little olive oil. Sprinkle with paprika, salt, pepper, and sesame seeds.

2. In a large skillet with coconut oil, sauté the fish, about 4-5 minutes on each side.

3. Serve over the lentil stew, with a lemon wedge on the side.

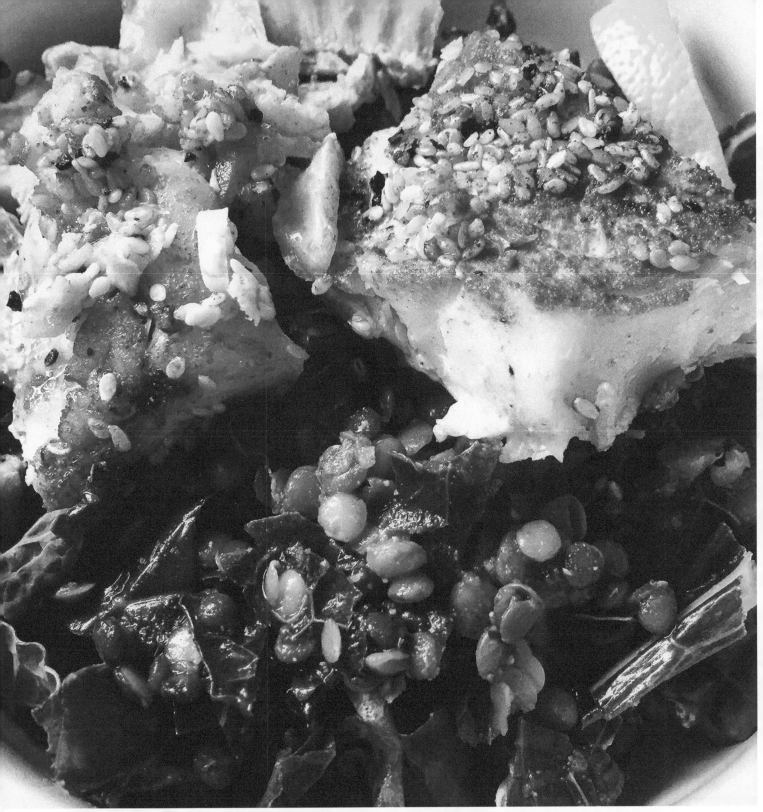

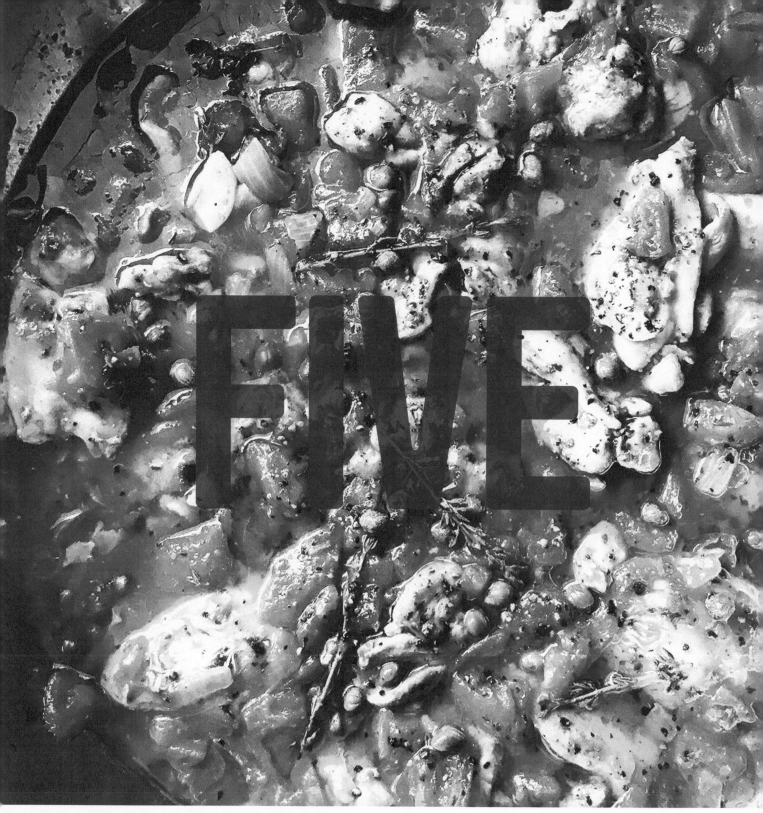

FIVE

CHICKEN
Kitchen MVP!

Everyone loves chicken! Chicken is by far the most popular choice for dinner for many people. It is naturally bland and absorbs easily any seasoning you put on it, and there are endless methods of preparing it. It is simple to prepare and readily available at any grocery store. Look for a certified-organic chicken to ensure a higher quality of chicken. I hope this section of my book will inspire you to discover and try a new chicken recipe that everyone would love.

WHOLE JERK CHICKEN

This chicken recipe is super-easy to prepare and offers lots of flavor from the rub, which takes a whole 5 minutes to prepare. This dish is one of our favorite chicken dinners.

HERE IS WHAT YOU NEED:

1 whole chicken, cleaned
  and patted dry

Rub:

¼ cup olive oil

2 tablespoon maple syrup

2 teaspoon paprika

1 teaspoon sea salt

½ teaspoon ground
  black pepper

½ teaspoon garlic powder

½ teaspoon onion powder

½ teaspoon dried thyme

¼ teaspoon ginger

¼ teaspoon cinnamon

¼ teaspoon allspice

Juice from 1 lime
  (save the fruit)

3 garlic cloves, halved

LET'S DO THIS:

1. Place the chicken in the center of a low-rimmed oven-safe dish lined with parchment paper or foil (for easy clean-up) with the breast facing up. Sprinkle sea salt all over the chicken and inside its cavity. Place the lime halves and garlic cloves inside the cavity and tie the chicken legs with kitchen twine.

2. Combine the rub ingredients and spread it all over the chicken and under the skin. Work with your hands for best results.

3. Roast at 375°F for 90 minutes. If the chicken is small, 1 hour will suffice. Let cool for a few minutes. Separate the chicken parts using kitchen shears, and serve.

Seeds for Thought... *For the best-tasting chicken, use ½ teaspoon sea salt per 1 pound of chicken! Salt helps season the meat and keep it moist.*

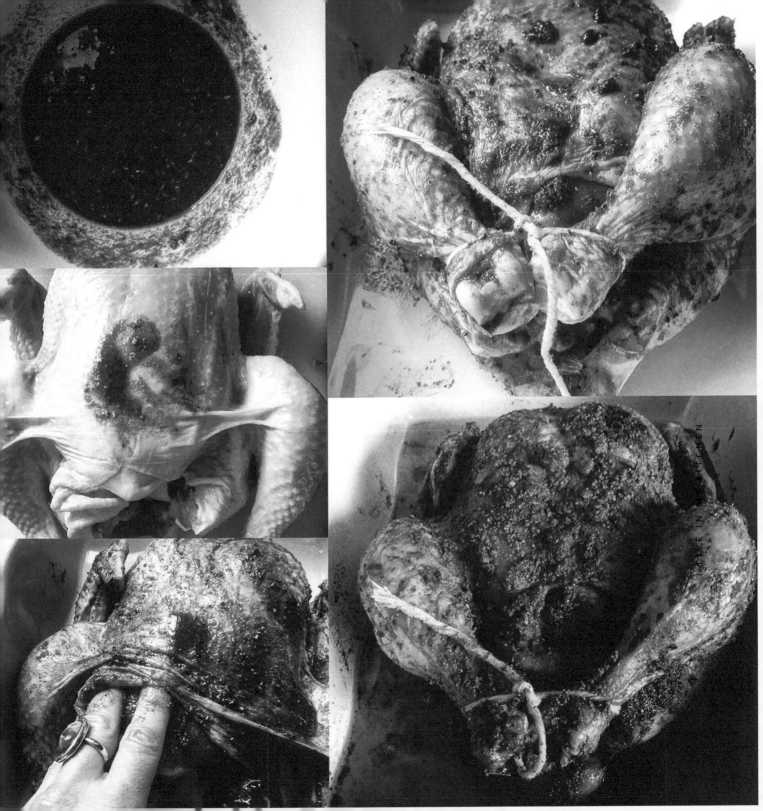

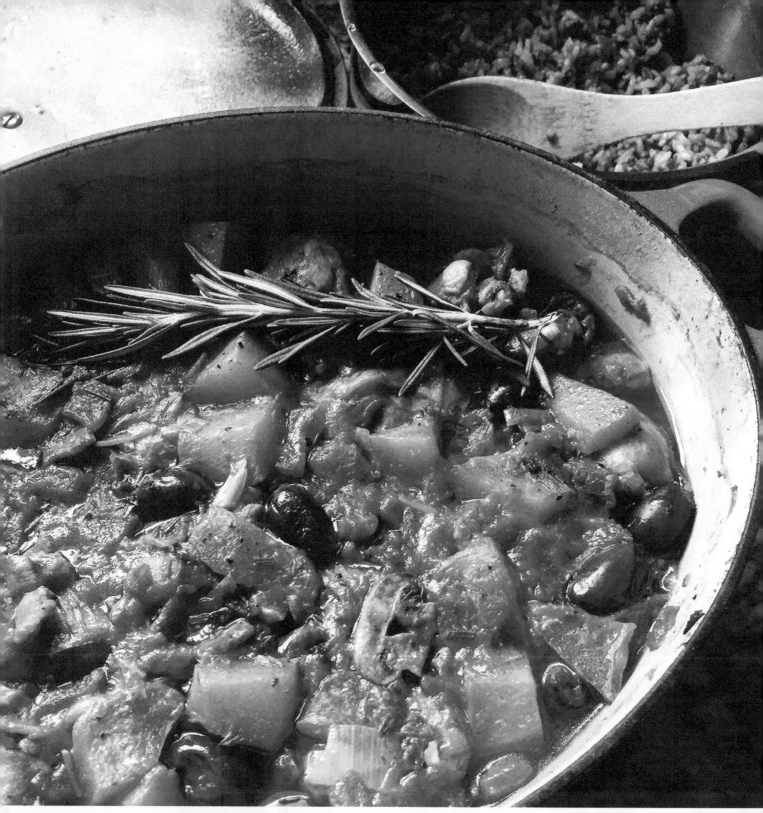

CHICKEN & BUTTERNUT SQUASH CACCIATORE

This dish is perfect for a cold and rainy day when all you want to do is curl up under the covers and eat homemade food. This dish will make your house smell good for hours. It is very easy to put together and will feed a family of 4 or 5 for two nights.

HERE IS WHAT YOU NEED:

3-4 tablespoons olive oil

1 onion, chopped

1 leek, chopped

4 pieces turkey bacon, chopped

1 stem rosemary, chopped

4 garlic cloves, chopped

6 boneless thighs

6 chicken legs, skin removed (or any combo of bone-in chicken)

1 lbs. butternut squash, cleaned and cubed

1 package sliced mushrooms (any variety), about 1 ½ cups total

1 cup good red wine (you can substitute with water or chicken stock)

1 can diced stewed tomatoes

1 small can tomato paste

10 Kalamta olives

Salt and pepper

LET'S DO THIS:

1. Place a heavy stove-to-oven pot on low-medium heat. Add all ingredients in the order they appear in 2 to 4-minute intervals, to allow them to cook a bit.

2. Bring the mixture to a light boil, then lower the heat to low and cover. Let simmer for 5 minutes, then transfer to a 375°F oven for 1 hour.

3. Serve over any sprouted or basmati rice. Yum!

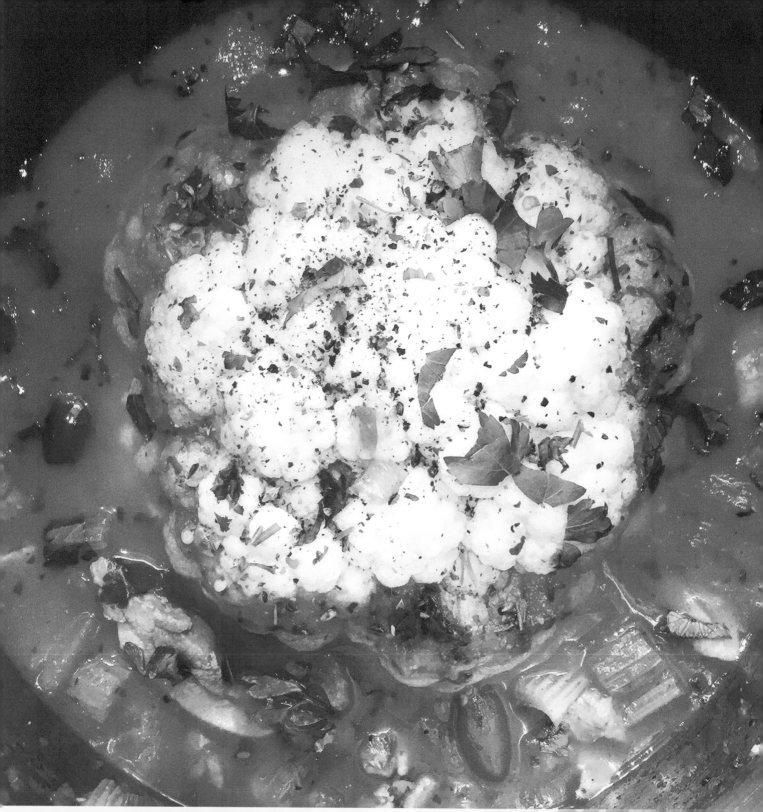

CAULIFLOWER & CHICKEN STEW

If you think cauliflower is boring, this recipe will prove you wrong! Thanks to its bland flavor, cauliflower will adapt to any seasoning and style of cooking. There are two versions for this recipe: one is vegetarian / vegan, and the other includes chicken breast in the sauce—so you can prepare what works best for you. Both versions are full of flavor and very satisfying.

HERE IS WHAT YOU NEED:

3-4 tablespoons olive oil

1 chopped onion

3 garlic cloves, crushed

4 celery stalks, sliced

1 head cauliflower

1 (15-ounces) jar organic marinara sauce

Equal amount of water

1 (14.2-ounces) can of crushed tomatoes

1 teaspoon garlic powder

1 teaspoon onion powder

½ teaspoon paprika

¼ teaspoon chili powder

A few sprinkles of dried oregano

½ cup pitted Kalamata olives

½ cup chopped parsley (optional: extra parsley, to garnish before serving)

2 tablespoons red wine vinegar

3-4 chicken breasts, cubed

LET'S DO THIS:

1. In a large pot, heat the oil on medium heat and add the onions, crushed garlic, and chopped celery. Sauté for 4-5 minutes.

2. Place the cauliflower in the middle of the pot. Circling around the cauliflower, pour in the marinara sauce, crushed tomatoes, and water. Continue to cook on medium heat. Make sure that 1" of the cauliflower is still above the sauce level.

3. Add the seasoning (including the vinegar and olives) to the sauce and stir gently.

4. For the chicken version, add the chicken cubes at this point. Bring to a gentle boil, lower the heat and cover the pot. Cook for 30 minutes or until the cauliflower is soft.

TRADITIONAL CHICKEN WITH ROOT VEGGIES

This is a traditional dish from my Mom's kitchen. I tweaked it a bit to fit my family's taste buds, so feel free to do the same. You can assemble it the night before, then pop it in the oven when you get home the next day. The ingredients are easy to find, and the recipe makes a very pretty presentation.

HERE IS WHAT YOU NEED:

4 chicken breasts (bone in)

6 chicken legs (or any combo of 10 chicken pieces you like, bone in)

2 lbs. tricolor carrots (or regular carrots), peeled and cut into big chunks

1 celery head, cleaned and cut into chunks

2 medium potatoes, cubed

1 parsnip, peeled and cut into chunks

2 onions cut into large pieces

¼ cup olive oil

½ lemon cut into wedges

1 whole garlic head cut in half horizontally

1-2 tablespoon cumin (no, it's not too much!)

1 ½ teaspoon salt

Freshly ground pepper

LET'S DO THIS:

1. Combine everything in a large and deep baking dish. Use your hands to toss everything well. Organize evenly in the pan.

2. At this stage, you can either bake it right away or store covered in the refrigerator for the next day. Bake covered at 375°F for 90 minutes.

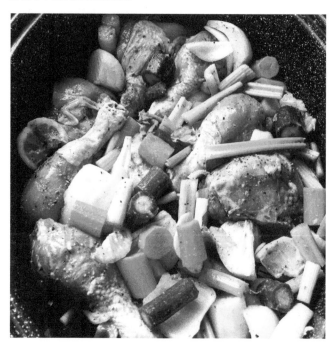

CHICKEN & POTATOES

Here is a very simple chicken dish with Middle Eastern flavors that everyone will love. The potatoes absorb the flavor of the chicken and seasonings. You will need a large baking dish with a lid, and you are ready to go!

HERE IS WHAT YOU NEED:

12 pieces of chicken, bone-in (remove the skin)

8-10 small potatoes, halfed

2 onions, chunks

1 garlic head cut in half (horizontally)

¼ cup olive oil

1 tablespoon cumin

1 tablespoon za'atar

1 teaspoon garlic powder

Optional: thyme or rosemary sprigs (or any fresh herbs you have on hand)

2-3 teaspoons sea salt

Freshly ground pepper

LET'S DO THIS:

1. Clean and pat the chicken dry.

2. Combine all of the ingredients in a large baking dish with a lid. Toss everything with your hands, making sure to arrange the mixture evenly in the dish.

3. Bake covered at 375°F for 1 hour and 15 minutes.

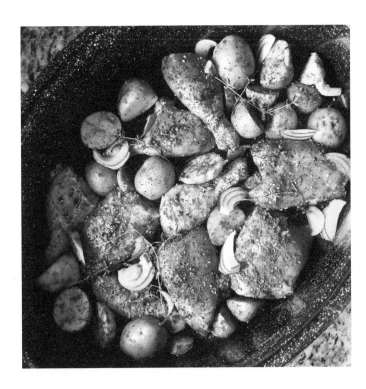

JUICY MIREPOIX CHICKEN

This is a colorful and juicy chicken dish. This recipe is made in a large skillet with a lid, which saves both clean up and cooking time. It can be done with any chicken parts, so pick the ones you and your family love most.

HERE IS WHAT YOU NEED:

6 chicken legs

4 boneless skinless chicken thighs (or any other 10 chicken parts)

¼ cup olive oil

1 onion, diced

4 carrots, chopped into coins

4 celery stalks, chopped small

5-6 garlic cloves, chopped

Salt and pepper

½ to 1 cup red wine (optional)

1 cup water

LET'S DO THIS:

1. In a large skillet, heat the olive oil on medium-low, and add the onions to sauté for 3-4 minutes until soft and golden. Add the carrots, celery and garlic and let them sauté lightly.

2. In the meantime, clean the chicken, pat it dry, and sprinkle it with salt and pepper. Add to the pan and sauté for a few minutes on each side.

3. Add the water and wine, sprinkle a little bit more salt, cover with a lid, and transfer to a 375°F oven. Bake for 30 minutes.

4. Serve over basmati white rice or quinoa, and enjoy the flavorful sauce of this dish.

5. Note: you can substitute the wine with water mixed with 3 tablespoons coconut aminos or organic soy sauce.

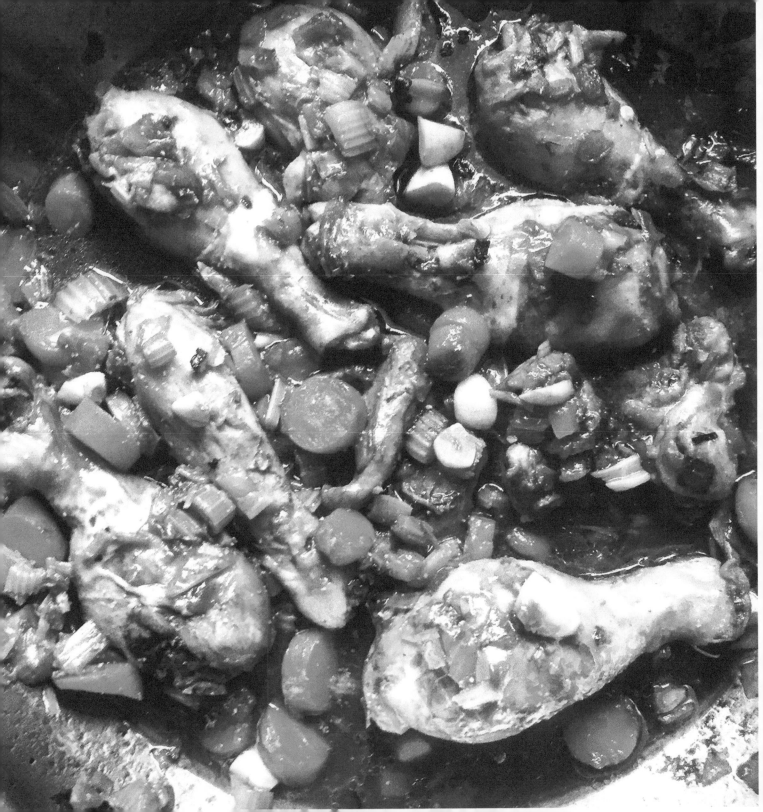

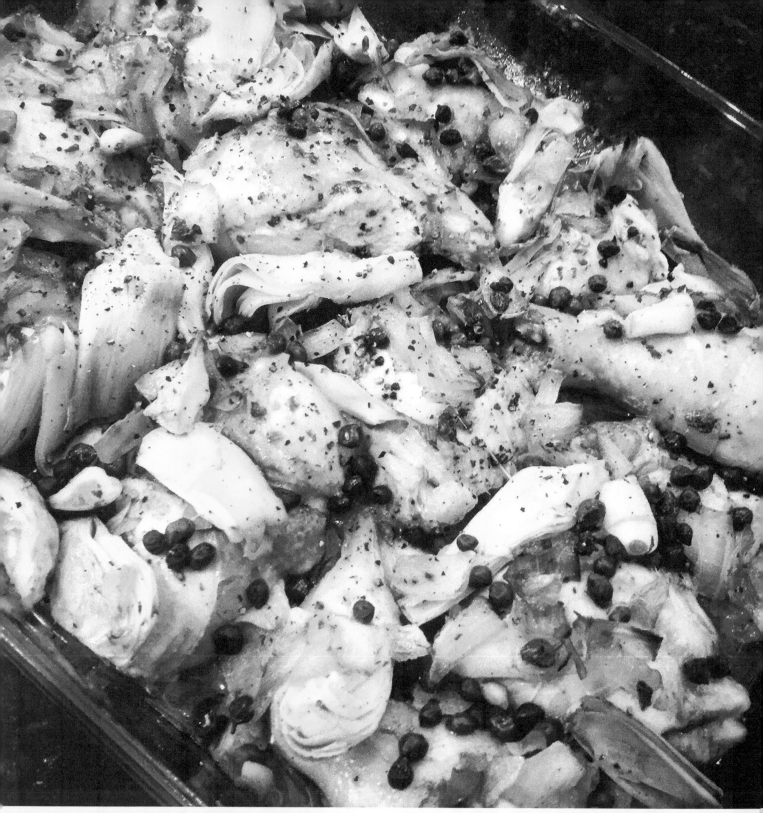

ARTICHOKE CHICKEN

This is another easy recipe that is great for both the middle of the week and special occasions—thanks to the artichokes, which give it a fancier look. Basic ingredients combine to make a moist, juicy chicken that everyone will love, even picky eaters. As with my other recipes, you can use any chicken parts—but keep in mind, boneless chicken may need a shorter cooking time. There are two ways to prepare this dish, and both result in a beautiful and tasty meal. If you are low on time, simply toss all of the ingredients (except the water) in a large bowl. Arrange in a baking dish, add the water to the sides of the chicken, and bake for 1 hour and 15 minutes. Or, follow the method below.

HERE IS WHAT YOU NEED:

10-12 chicken pieces, bone-in

¼ cup olive oil

1 tablespoon coconut oil

1 onion, chopped

3 garlic cloves, crushed

1 can artichokes hearts (halved)

3 tablespoons capers, rinsed

4-5 sprigs thyme (fresh or dried—you can also use oregano or rosemary)

1 cup water

Salt and pepper to taste

LET'S DO THIS:

1. Clean the chicken and sprinkle with salt, pepper, and olive oil.

2. Using medium heat, preheat the pan with 3 tablespoons of olive oil. Sear the chicken pieces gently on both sides. Set them into a large baking dish.

3. In the same pan, add the coconut oil and sauté the onions, garlic, and artichokes hearts until golden. Spread on the chicken.

4. Add the water, capers and a dash of salt to the pan, stir gently, and scrape up all of the chicken leftovers from Step 2.

5. Transfer the liquid mixture into the dish, but not directly onto the chicken. Sprinkle the chicken with thyme, and bake at 375°F for 1 hour.

6. Before serving, drizzle 1-2 tablespoons olive oil all over the chicken to intensify the flavor.

WHOLE ZA'ATAR CHICKEN

This chicken recipe is another staple in my house nowadays. It takes less than 5 minutes to prepare, and the result is crispy on the outside, and juicy and flavorful within. There are three ways you can make this recipe. You can use a whole chicken that has its legs tied with twine. Alternatively, you can use a flattened whole chicken; using kitchen scissors, slice along the back, then lay the chicken out flat, breast side up, some butchers can do this for you. Lastly, you can use cut-up chicken pieces; spread them out evenly on a baking sheet with ¼" space between each piece. Whichever method you choose, you will end up with delicious chicken everyone will ask for seconds.

HERE IS WHAT YOU NEED:

1 whole organic chicken (or chicken pieces), washed and patted completely dry, so the seasoning doesn't wash off

½ cup olive oil

⅓ cup za'atar spice

Garlic head, cut in half horizontally

Salt and pepper

LET'S DO THIS:

1. Line a roasting pan with small rim with parchment paper or foil.

2. Place the chicken in the middle of the pan, sprinkle it with salt and pepper, and place the garlic underneath it.

3. Mix the oil with the za'atar in a small bowl. Spread the paste all over the chicken and if possible, insert some beneath the skin. Use your hands for best results.

4. Bake at 375° F for 75 minutes uncovered and discover a delightful chicken that is crispy on the outside, juicy on the inside.

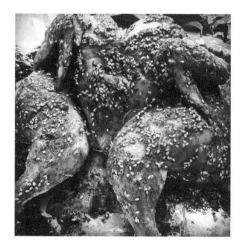

Seeds for Thought... Za'atar is a Middle Eastern spice blend made from dried thyme, sumac, sesame seeds, and sometimes salt and other spices. You can find it in health food stores or markets, or seek it out online. Za'atar is terrific in salads with olive oil and lemon. You can also add it to olive oil to create a dip; sprinkle it over pizza; or use it to season any fish.

CHICKEN PICCATA

What a fancy name for a super simple dish! Piccata is an Italian word meaning "larded," cooking using butter or oil. While piccata sauces often contain wine, here, we are allowing the spices to speak for themselves. This dish is bursting with flavor and creates a nice sauce you can drizzle over rice or quinoa.

HERE IS WHAT YOU NEED:

4-5 chicken breasts (it they are too big, split them in half)

2 tablespoons coconut oil

1-2 shallots, diced (or 1 small onion)

1 cup chicken stock (or vegetable stock, or water)

2 garlic cloves crushed

3 tablespoons capers (rinsed)

1 teaspoon dried thyme

1 teaspoon dried oregano

Lemon juice (typically half a lemon)

Salt and pepper

LET'S DO THIS:

1. Sauté the chicken breasts in a large skillet on both sides, about 3-4 minutes per side, until golden. Transfer the chicken to a plate.

2. Add 2 tablespoons oil to the pan and sauté the shallots. Add the garlic, capers, chicken stock, seasonings, lemon juice, and bring to a light boil.

3. Add the chicken back into the skillet and cover. Cook for another 10-15 minutes. Garnish with thin lemon slices.

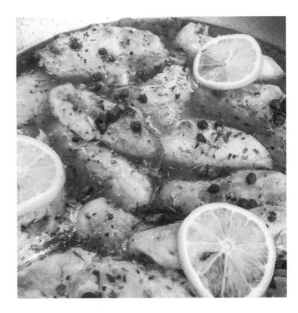

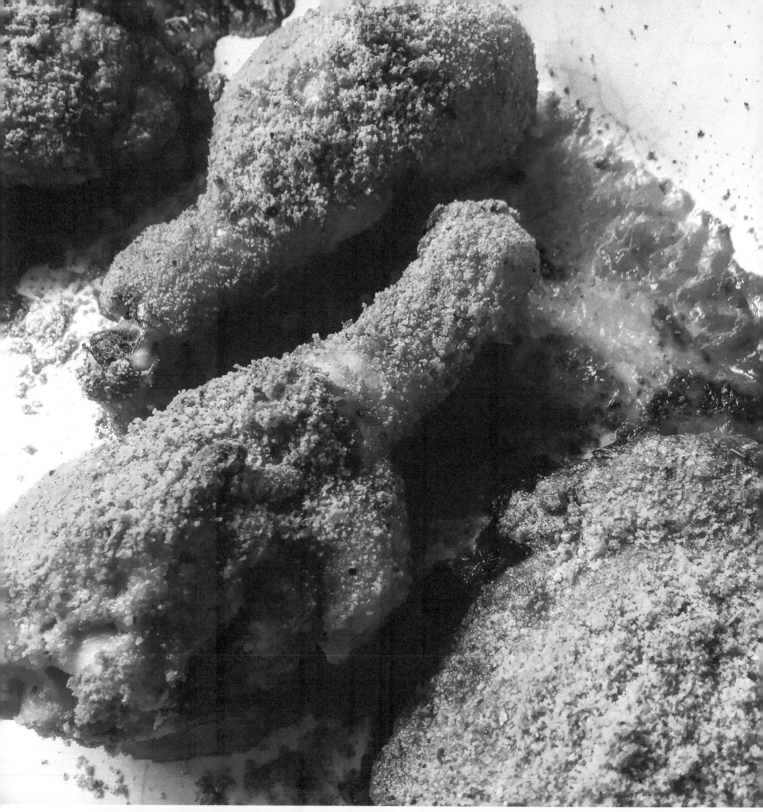

FAVORITE SHAKE & BAKE

This dish is definitely a staple in my house; I hope it will be in yours, too! It is healthy and very simple to make. I use different parts of chicken each time, so please feel free to do the same, with or without bones. Bake for one hour if you are using bone-in chicken, and for 45 minutes if using boneless chicken.

HERE IS WHAT YOU NEED:

8-12 pieces of chicken, skinless

In a Ziploc® bag combine:
1 cup almond meal
1 tablespoon paprika
1 teaspoon dried oregano
½ teaspoon garlic powder
Salt and pepper
Pinch chili powder (optional)

LET'S DO THIS:

1. Moisten the chicken pieces with a scant amount of water.

2. Drop two pieces of chicken at a time into the Ziploc® bag and shake to coat. Make sure you keep the top part of the bag tightly closed.

3. Arrange the chicken, leaving about ½" space between pieces, on parchment paper or an oven-safe ceramic dish and bake at 375°F. Bake for one hour for chicken with bones or 45 minutes if using boneless chicken.

SHAWARMA CHICKEN

Shawarma is a very popular fast food in Israel. It is sold in small kiosks that specialize in making shawarma and falafel, since both are served in a pita with assorted chopped salads, pickles, hummus, and tahini. Practically a whole meal in pita bread, delicious!! Shawarma is typically made of lamb meat or a mix of lamb and chicken stacked on a large upright skewer, with pieces of lamb fat placed alongside the meat for flavor. If you can't make it to a shawarma stand anytime soon, try this recipe instead; it will get you close enough to the original...

HERE IS WHAT YOU NEED:

6-8 skinless boneless thighs (dark meat is better, but you can still use white meat), clean, patted dry and sliced into strips

2 tablespoons cumin

1 teaspoon paprika

6 garlic cloves, minced

1 lemon, juice only

¼ cup olive oil

Salt and pepper

2 tablespoons coconut or olive oil, for cooking

LET'S DO THIS:

1. Place all of the ingredients in a bowl and mix well. Make sure the seasonings are distributed evenly. It is best to let the chicken marinade in the seasoning for 2 hours or overnight.

2. In a skillet, warm the oil on medium heat, add the chicken, and let sear well on all sides. Don't turn the meat over too much; simply let it sear on one side, then flip it to the other. Spread out the strips each time you toss and flip to ensure the meat is cooked evenly.

3. While the chicken is cooking, chop tomatoes, cucumbers, parsley, olive oil, salt and pepper and combine to make a quick Israeli salad.

4. Serve the chicken with a side of pita bread, hummus, or tahini, and the salad, for a complete Israeli experience.

Seeds for Thought... Spices are crucial for making delicious dishes. Invest a small fortune in high quality and fresh spices to transform boring foods to flavorful and memorable dishes.

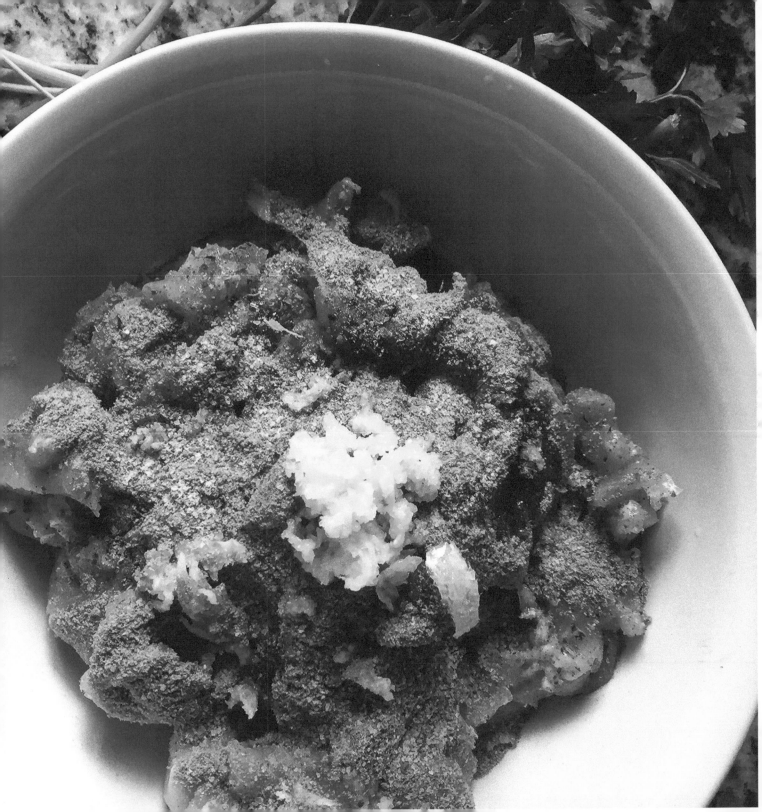

FANCY CHICKEN PAELLA

This version of chicken paella offers a rainbow of seasonings and aromas from the spanish cuisine. It is a one-dish meal everyone will love and ask for more .

HERE IS WHAT YOU NEED:

¼ cup olive oil

1-1 ½ lbs. boneless and skinless chicken pieces

1 onion, chopped

1½ cups chopped red/yellow/green peppers, any combo

1 (14.5-ounce) can stewed tomatoes, cubed

2 cups organic basmati rice (rinsed and drained)

4 cups water

1 bag of frozen or fresh peas

3 teaspoons paprika

Salt and pepper

2 pinches of saffron

1 lemon cut in half (for serving)

LET'S DO THIS:

1. Sprinkle paprika, salt, and pepper on the chicken. In a large skillet on medium heat, warm the oil, and sauté the chicken tenders. Move the tenders to a plate.

2. Add the chopped onions and peppers to the pan, and sauté lightly. Add the tomatoes and saffron, stir, and let everything cook for a few minutes. Place the chicken back into the pan.

3. Add the water and rice and stir lightly on medium-high heat. Once the water starts to boil, lower the heat, and cover. Simmer for 20 minutes.

4. Uncover. Spread the peas over the chicken and rice, cover, and simmer for 15 minutes.

5. Serve the paella with wedge of lemon to squeeze all over.

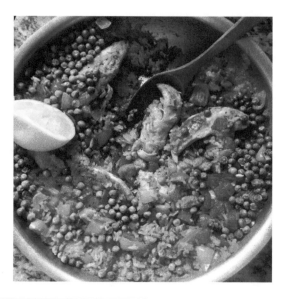

CHICKEN STIR FRY

This is a great recipe for a mid-week fix. If you have a few minutes the night before to prepare the vegetables, it will be super-easy and quick to cook the next day. Nowadays, you can find pre-cut vegetables in most supermarkets; stock up to make your cooking life much easier. This recipe calls for coconut aminos, which is a substitution for soy sauce. It tastes very similar to soy sauce but is made out of coconut tree sap.

HERE IS WHAT YOU NEED:

4 tablespoons coconut oil

1 onion

1-2 peppers in different colors

2 crushed garlic cloves

1 sweet potato

2-3 bok choy

1 (4-ounce) package mushrooms (2 cups)

1 lb. chicken tenders (or any other parts of boneless chicken)

Salt and pepper

3 tablespoons coconut aminos or organic soy sauce

Handful chopped cashews

Sesame seeds (optional)

LET'S DO THIS:

1. Cut all vegetables into strips. Do the same with the chicken.

2. Use medium heat to warm the oil in a large skillet and start sautéing the vegetables, adding them to the skillet in the order they are listed. Stir after each addition.

3. In a separate skillet on medium heat, sauté the chicken with 1 tablespoon coconut oil until fully cooked. Sprinkle sesame seeds all over the chicken. Suggestion: cook the vegetables and the chicken simultaneously.

4. Transfer the chicken to the vegetables. Sprinkle with salt, pepper, and coconut aminos. Stir and cook everything together for two more minutes on medium-low heat. Sprinkle chopped cashews on top for some crunch.

5. Serve over basmati rice.

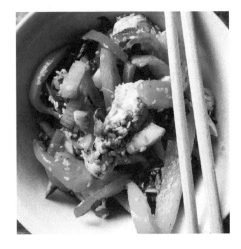

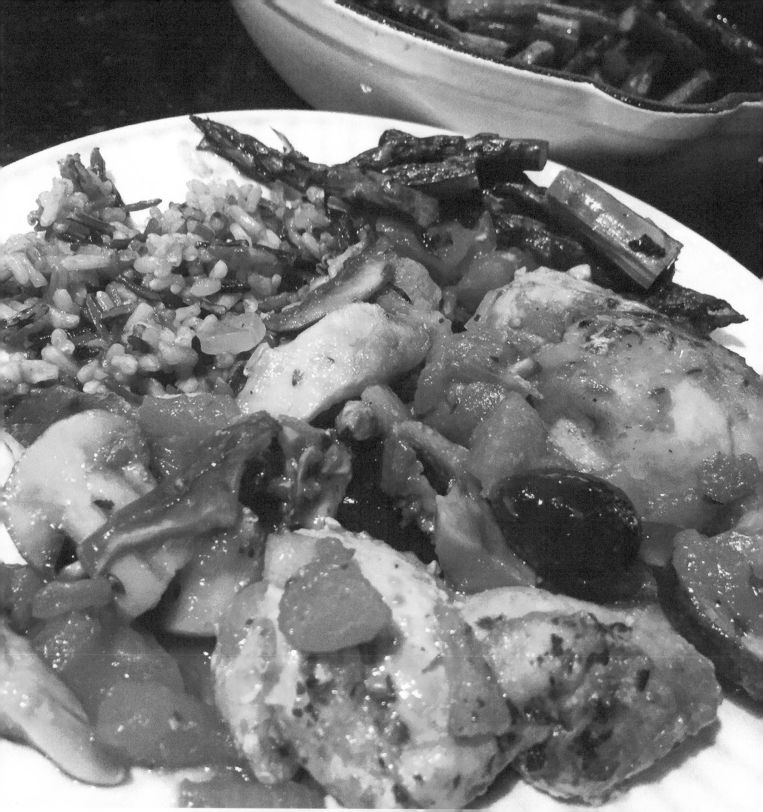

MUSHROOMS & CHICKEN FEST

This is a great mid-week dish with a winning combination of flavors from the chicken, shitake mushrooms, and tomatoes. The chicken comes out so juicy and moist that everyone will lick their fingers.

HERE IS WHAT YOU NEED:

1 large onion, diced

2 tablespoons coconut oil

10 skinless boneless thighs (or any other chicken pieces—bone-in works well, too)

1 (4-ounces) package bella mushrooms, sliced

A handful shitake mushrooms, sliced (optional: use more mushrooms or a different type)

1 (14-ounces) can organic diced tomatoes

1 cup water

4 garlic cloves, crushed

1 teaspoon dried thyme

1 teaspoon dried oregano

1 tablespoon apple cider vinegar

5 black olives, pitted

Salt and pepper

LET'S DO THIS:

1. Using a large skillet, sauté the onions for 3-4 minutes. Add the mushrooms and continue to sauté for another 10 minutes until both onions and mushrooms are caramelized with a golden-brown color.

2. Make room for the chicken by pushing the onions and the mushrooms to the sides of the pan. Add the chicken and sauté for a few minutes on each side.

3. Add the tomatoes, water, garlic and seasonings and bring to a boil. Add the olives. Lower the heat and simmer for 5 minutes, covered.

4. Transfer to a 375°F oven and bake for 20 minutes, uncovered. If using bone in chicken, bake for 40 minutes.

Optional: After Step 2, transfer the chicken and the mushrooms to a large baking dish. Add the tomatoes, water, and seasonings. Bake for 375°F for 45 minutes, uncovered.

CHICKEN PAELLA

This is a quick version of the popular Spanish dish. The key to making it easy to prepare is to use a large skillet with a lid; it saves time for both cooking and cleaning up! This dish is perfect for the middle of the week or for entertaining, because it is beautifully presented and great for sharing.

HERE IS WHAT YOU NEED:

3 chicken breasts or 6 skinless boneless thighs (chopped into 1"x1" pieces)

4 tablespoons olive oil, for step 1

1 onion, diced

2 carrots, cut into chunks

1-2 celery stalks, cut into chunks

1 teaspoon paprika

Salt and pepper

2 tablespoons olive oil, for step 3

1½ cups organic basmati rice (rinsed and drained)

3 cups water

½ teaspoon saffron

½ cup sun-dried tomatoes

LET'S DO THIS:

1. Heat the oil in a skillet on the stove, using medium heat. Add the onions, carrots and celery, and sauté for 5 minutes.

2. In the meantime, sprinkle the chicken pieces with paprika, salt, and pepper.

3. Move the vegetables to the side of the pan. Add 2 tablespoons olive oil to the middle of the pan, and sauté the chicken. Let it sear for about 2 minutes on each side.

4. Add the rice to the skillet and mix everything together. Add the water, saffron and sun-dried tomatoes. Mix gently. Bring to a boil, lower the heat to low, and cover for 20-30 minutes. Uncover, add salt and pepper if needed, and make sure the rice is done. Turn off heat and let sit covered for 5 minutes.

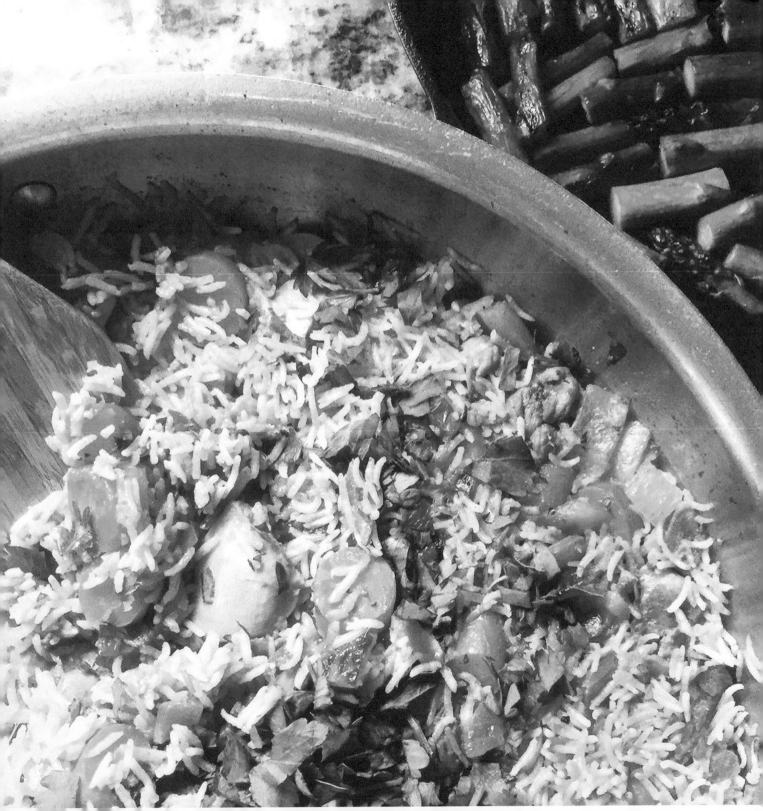

SIZZLING CHICKEN THIGHS

Skinless boneless chicken thighs are not only juicy and tender, but they are also packed with more nutrients than the white parts. They cook fast and can be used in an array of recipes. Keep a package in the freezer for a last-minute meal fix. Simply, take out of the freezer in the morning, leave them in the sink to defrost; they will be ready to prepare by the afternoon.

HERE IS WHAT YOU NEED:

6-10 boneless skinless chicken thighs (or breasts)

Marinade:

¼ cup olive oil

1 tablespoon cumin

1 teaspoon garlic powder

1 teaspoon paprika

Lime juice (or lemon juice)

2 garlic cloves, minced

Salt and pepper

LET'S DO THIS:

1. Mix the marinade in a small bowl and combine with the chicken in a Ziploc® bag. Squeeze the thighs through the bag, to make sure they are fully covered with the seasonings. This also tenderizes the chicken. Let the chicken marinate for at least an hour and up to a day in the refrigerator.

2. Heat the grill to 400°F or use a skillet on the stove on medium-high, and grill / sear each side for approximately 4-5 minutes.

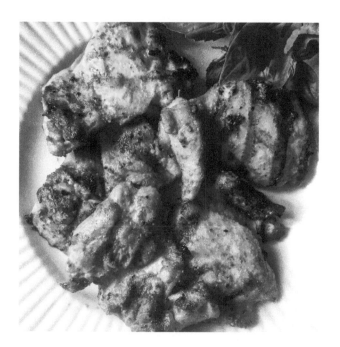

CHICKEN CURRY

If you like Indian food, this one is for you! The chicken and cauliflower absorb the wonderful flavors of the Indian seasonings and the result is a very satisfying and delicious dish.

HERE IS WHAT YOU NEED:

3 tablespoons coconut oil

1 onion, diced

1 cauliflower head, broken into small florets

6 boneless skinless chicken thighs cubed (or 4 chicken breasts cubed)

½ lemon, juice only

1" ginger, peeled and thinly sliced

1 can (14-ounce) light coconut milk

½ cup water

½ teaspoon of each: turmeric, curry, cumin, cinnamon, and salt

LET'S DO THIS:

1. Beginning with the oil, add all of the ingredients listed above to a large skillet on medium heat. Add one ingredient at a time, with a two-minute intervals in between, to allow each item to cook thoroughly.

2. After everything has been added to the skillet, bring to a gentle boil, lower the heat and simmer covered for 20-30 minutes.

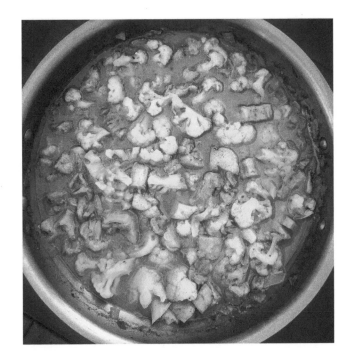

OLIVES & TOMATO CHICKEN

This dish bursts with colors and flavors. Use a large pan with a lid, which will save you time and cleanup—you can even use it to store leftovers, for easy reheating the next day. Don't let the list of spices to intimidate you, most likely you have them all in your kitchen, and if you are missing one or two spices, it will still taste wonderful.

HERE IS WHAT YOU NEED:

4 tablespoons olive oil

1 medium onion, chopped

3 minced garlic cloves

1.5 lbs. chicken tenders (or chicken breast cut into chunks)

5-6 mini peppers, cleaned and quartered, or 1 red pepper, diced

1 (14.5-ounce) can fire-roasted organic tomatoes (or another variety of cubed stewed tomato, or 3 fresh tomatoes cubed)

1 teaspoon paprika

1 teaspoon cumin

1 teaspoon garlic powder

1 teaspoon dried oregano

Sea salt and pepper

Cayenne pepper, just a pinch

15 pitted Kalamata olives

Chopped parsley, for garnish

LET'S DO THIS:

1. In a large skillet on medium-low heat, add the oil. Add the ingredients above in the order they are listed. Be sure to stir before you add each one.

2. Bring to a gentle boil. Lower the heat, cover and simmer for about 20 minutes.

Optional: Garnish with parsley and serve over cauliflower rice.

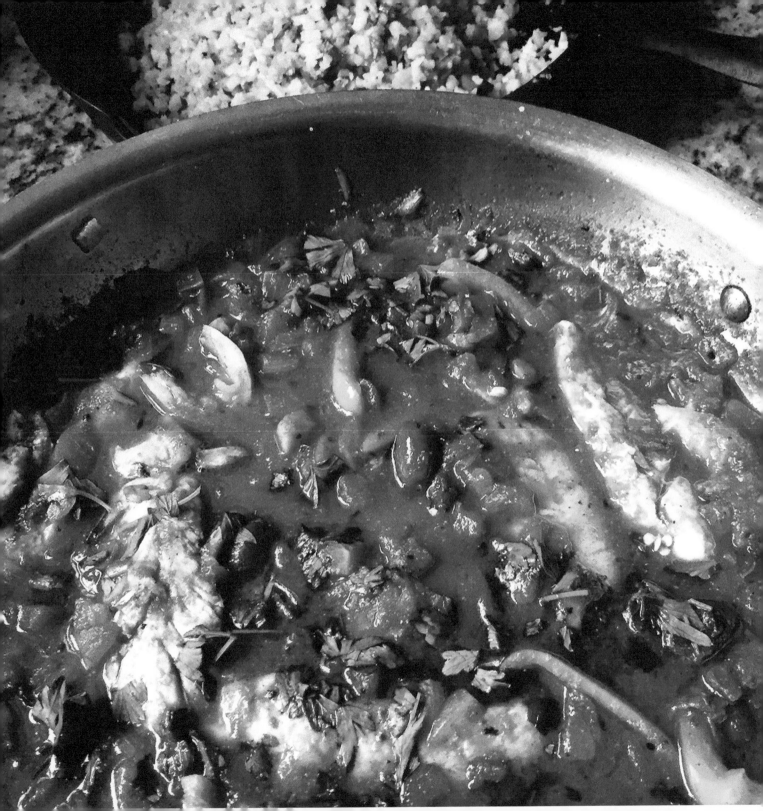

MIDDLE EASTERN GRILLED CHICKEN

This super-easy recipe for chicken can be cooked on the grill, in the oven, or in a cast iron skillet on the stove. It uses fresh herbs and lemon rind, which combine to give the chicken deep aromas and true Middle Eastern taste. Let the chicken marinate for at least one hour and up to one day, so it can absorb the full range of flavors.

HERE IS WHAT YOU NEED:

8-10 chicken thighs or breasts (skinless and boneless)

Marinade:

1 lemon, juice

1 lemon, grated rind

2 cups of finely chopped fresh herbs, like parsley, thyme, and oregano

⅓ cup olive oil

1 tablespoon cumin

½ teaspoon sea salt

Fresh ground pepper

8 garlic cloves, minced

2 teaspoons sumac (optional)

LET'S DO THIS:

1. Combine all the marinade ingredients in a large bowl. Add the chicken to the marinade and mix thoroughly. Let the chicken marinate in the fridge for at least an hour and up to 24 hours.

2. Line a cookie sheet with foil and lay the chicken flat. Positioning the tray about ⅓ of the way down from the broiler, broil for 15 minutes or until golden brown, take out and turn to the other side, broil for another 5 minutes. Or grill at 400°F, for approximately 5 minutes each side. Alternately, using a cast iron skillet on medium-high heat, sear the chicken about 5 minutes on each side.

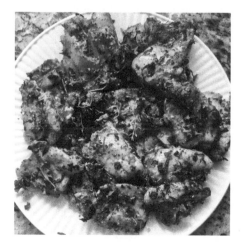

PEACHY CHICKEN

This is a great recipe to enjoy peaches in season. An old recipe that calls for peach preserves inspired me to create this one with a few tweaks. I removed the sugar and additives, but kept the rich taste of the peaches. It is very easy to put together and will fool everyone into thinking you spent all day in the kitchen!

HERE IS WHAT YOU NEED:

2 onions, slivered

2 tablespoons coconut oil

8 pieces of bone-in chicken (boneless pieces will work, as well)

Salt and pepper

2 sprigs each of thyme and oregano

3 yellow peaches, cubed small

6-8 garlic cloves, halved

LET'S DO THIS:

1. Sauté the onions with the oil in a large skillet on medium heat, until caramelized to a deep golden brown. This might take about 10 minutes.

2. In the meantime, clean the chicken, pat it dry, and place it in a baking dish. Sprinkle salt and pepper, fresh herbs, and garlic halves all over.

3. Spread the caramelized onions on top of the chicken and top with the cubed peaches. Sprinkle a bit more sea salt and pepper on top.

4. Cover loosely with foil and bake at 400°F for 1 hour. Uncover and continue baking for another 15 minutes.

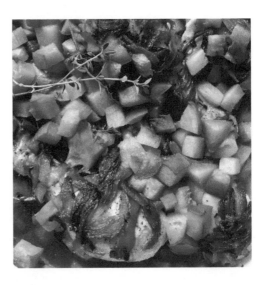

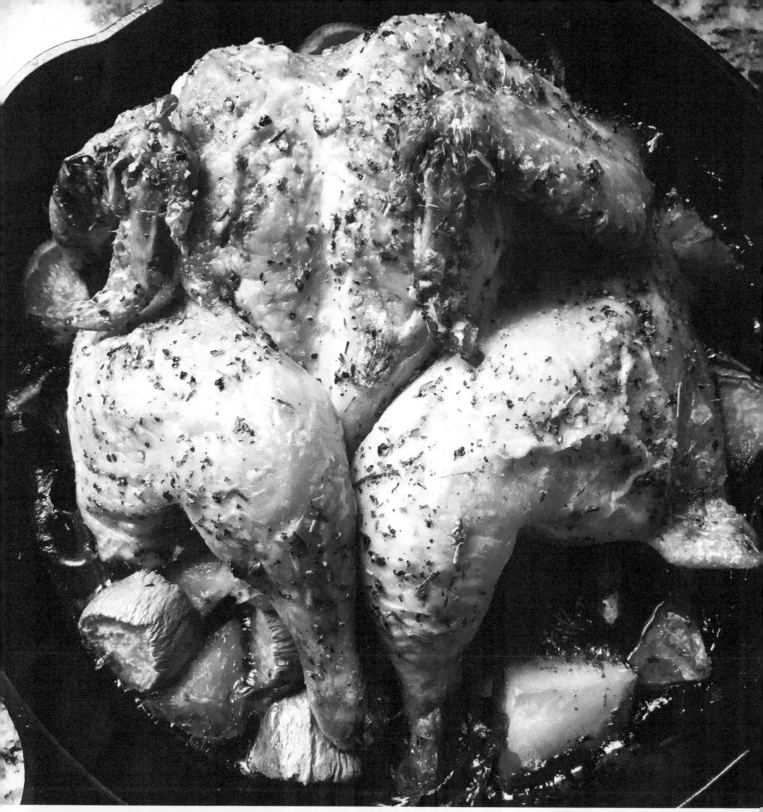

CITRUS ROASTED CHICKEN

The citrus aromas and flavors merge perfectly with the chicken and vegetables in this fabulous recipe. The chicken comes out moist and flavorful while your house smells delicious.

HERE IS WHAT YOU NEED:

1 whole organic chicken, split from the back

1 onion, chopped

1 sweet potato, chunks

1 regular potato, chunks

1 orange, skin on, cubed

1 head of garlic cut in half horizontally

1 teaspoon sea salt

Seasoning Blend:

⅓ cup olive oil

1 tablespoon dried thyme (or any combination of dried thyme, rosemary, and oregano)

¼ teaspoon orange rind

1 teaspoon sea salt

Ground black pepper

LET'S DO THIS:

1. In a cast iron skillet or any stove to oven dish, layer the garlic, potatoes, onion and orange.

2. Combine the seasoning blend in a small bowl.

3. Clean and pat the chicken dry. Sprinkle with sea salt all over the skin and cavity. Place it on top of the vegetables, tucking the legs inwards. Spread the seasoning blend all over the chicken and under the skin. Let it drip on the vegetables at the bottom.

4. Place the skillet on the stove on medium heat for about 5-10 minutes. Let the vegetables sear lightly.

5. Transfer to a 375°F oven and bake for an hour and a half uncovered. Let it cool for 10-15 minutes before serving.

JAMAICAN STYLE CHICKEN

This recipe can be done with a whole flat chicken or using bone-in chicken pieces. Either way, the chicken has to be cleaned and patted dry, to ensure better roasting. The chicken will emerge juicy on the inside and crispy on the outside.

HERE IS WHAT YOU NEED:

1 whole chicken (or cut into pieces)

1 head of garlic cut in half horizontally

Seasoning Blend:

2 teaspoon paprika

1 teaspoon cumin

½ teaspoon onion powder

½ teaspoon garlic powder

½ teaspoon dried oregano

⅓ cup olive oil

¼ teaspoon cinnamon

1 lime, juice only

Salt and pepper

Pinch nutmeg

Pinch cayenne pepper

LET'S DO THIS:

1. Clean the chicken, pat it dry, sprinkle sea salt on the cavity and place in the middle of a cookie sheet lined with foil or parchment paper, skin side up. Place the two garlic halves under the chicken.

2. Combine the seasonings blend and spread all over the chicken, including beneath the skin. Use your hands for best results.

3. Bake at 375°F for 90 minutes. If using chicken pieces, bake for one hour.

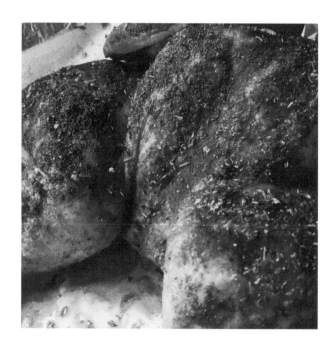

PAPRIKA CHICKEN

This recipe is just a spin on a dish my mom used to make with oil, paprika, salt, and pepper. It is the perfect example of how a simple combination of spices can turn a boring chicken to a flavorful and colorful dish. It is better to leave the chicken in the marinade for an hour or more, but it will still be tasty if you are short on time.

HERE IS WHAT YOU NEED:

1 lb. skinless, boneless chicken thighs (or chicken breast cut into large chunks)

1-2 tablespoons coconut oil

Marinade:

1 heaping tablespoon paprika

½ teaspoon smoked paprika

Pinch cayenne pepper

½ teaspoon garlic powder

3-4 garlic cloves, minced

¼ cup olive oil

Salt and pepper

LET'S DO THIS:

1. Mix all the seasonings (except for the coconut oil) to create a marinade.

2. Place the chicken in a large bowl and mix it with the marinade using two wooden spoons until the chicken is well coated. Cover and leave in the refrigerator for at least an hour or overnight.

3. When ready to cook the chicken, heat the coconut oil in a large skillet. Sear the chicken for about 4 minutes on each side. Lower the heat to very low and cook for another 10 minutes. Sprinkle with parsley or kale leaves before serving.

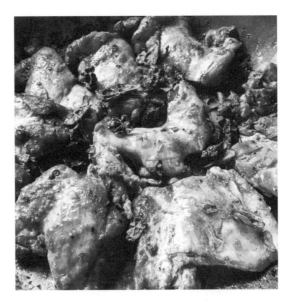

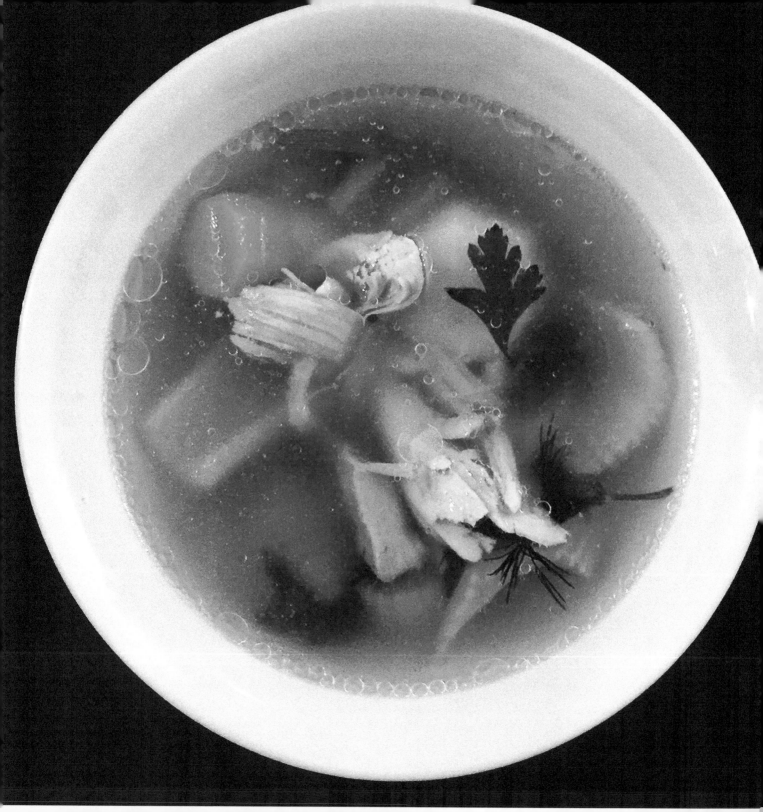

CHICKEN SOUP

———

Nothing says "home" like the aroma of chicken soup that has been cooking on the stove for hours. It reminds me so much of my childhood and my Mom's kitchen. It also brings back memories of family meals, holidays, and love. Although some call chicken soup "the Jewish Penicillin," many cultures share a love for this nourishing and comforting food. The long cooking process dissolves nutrients from the chicken bones, making the soup quite restorative and healing. A large pot of soup will keep in the refrigerator up to ten days so you and the family can enjoy a warm bowl of soup for days. If I have too much soup left, I store some in a mason jar and freeze it for later use.

For many years, I have experimented with soup stock powders, trying to enhance the flavor of the soup. But the truth is, you don't need any prepackaged powders to make a flavorful soup, the vegetables and the herbs are the essence of a flavorful chicken soup.

HERE IS WHAT YOU NEED:
Use these quantities below as a guide:

10 pieces of bone-in chicken, skin removed

1 whole celery head, cleaned and chopped into 2" chunks

2 lbs. carrots, peeled and chopped into 2" chunks

1 onion

1 bunch parsley, rinsed and cut in half

1 bunch dill, rinsed and cut in half

2 parsnips, peeled and chopped to big chunks

1 turnip, peeled and halved

3 tablespoons sea salt

Freshly ground pepper

1 teaspoon turmeric (mainly for color)

Large soup pot with a lid

LET'S DO THIS:

1. Combine everything in a large pot filled with water and place on the stove at high heat. Bring to a boil. Lower the heat to low and cover. Simmer for 3-4 hours.

2. Let the soup cool slightly. At this point you can either remove the chicken and transfer it to a separate dish, or remove the bones and return the chicken meat to the pot.

3. Remove the parsley, dill, parsnip and turnip from the pot and discard, as they have done their job.

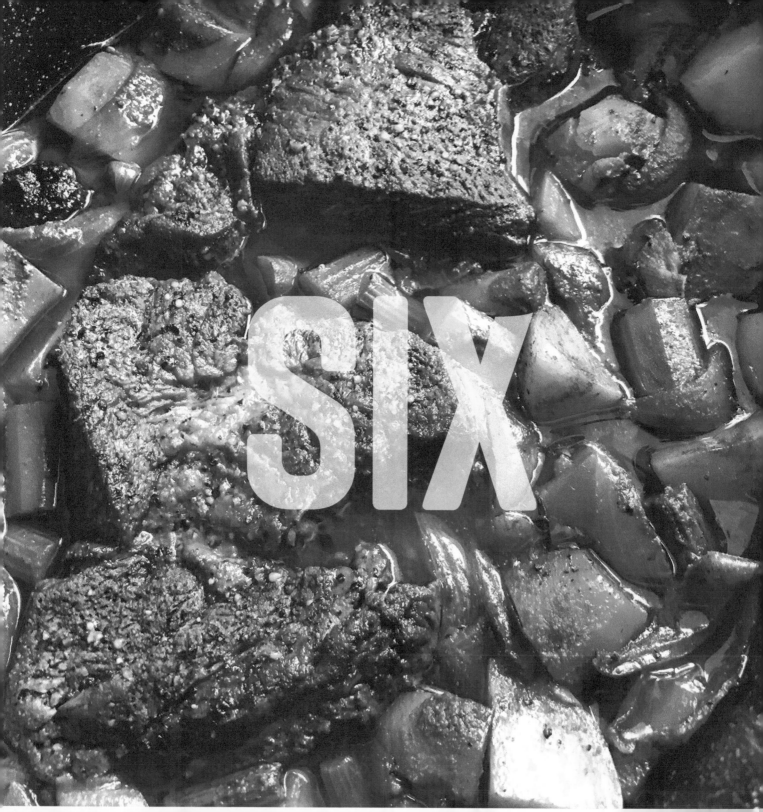

BEEF & LAMB
Sizzling!

Sometimes you just crave a juicy piece meat! Make sure to buy the best quality meat you can get your hands on, and enjoy the rich flavors and abundance of nutrients that red meat offers.

CRANBERRY & ONION BRISKET

This is a staple in my house for special occasions and holidays. Everyone goes for seconds and I rarely have any leftovers. The original recipe used canned cranberry sauce and powdered onion soup, both of which I have transformed into a cleaner version. It has the same rich flavors but without the artificial ingredients. It is best to prepare ahead of time, to avoid the messy step of slicing the meat on the day you are hosting the dinner.

HERE IS WHAT YOU NEED:

5-6 lbs. first-cut brisket, cleaned by the butcher

1 bag (or 2 cups) dried cranberries, soaked in hot water for a half hour

4 onions, chopped into thin slices

4 tablespoons coconut or olive oil

2 teaspoons sea salt

Black pepper

½ cup coconut aminos

½ cup water

Heavy-duty, large-size foil
Roasting pan
Skillet

LET'S DO THIS:

1. In a large skillet on medium heat, sauté the onions with the oil until golden brown and caramelized. Turn the heat to low.

2. Drain the cranberries and add them to the skillet with the onions. Add the coconut aminos, salt and pepper, and water and mix well until thoroughly combined. Turn off the heat.

3. Clear an area on your kitchen counter. Cut 3 long pieces of heavy-duty foil and lay them one on top of another, with the second layer crossing the first, and the third layer in the same direction as the first.

4. Pat the brisket dry and sprinkle sea salt all over it.

5. Pour half of the cranberry mixture into the middle of the top piece of tin foil. Place the brisket on top. Pour the rest of the mixture on top of the brisket and spread to cover the meat.

6. Start wrapping the brisket with the foil. Hold the piece of foil directly under the brisket, match the two ends, and fold at the edges to seal. Seal the sides as much as possible, then do the same with the other pieces of tin foil. The goal is to create a "pocket" in which the brisket can cook, so try to leave some space around the brisket, but seal the edges of the foil so the sauce will not escape. Once you have folded all three pieces of foil and the pocket is sealed, poke a hole with a sharp knife to release steam during cooking.

7. Place the "pocket" in a large roasting pan with a lid. Bake at 450°F for 30 minutes. Lower the heat to 300°F and roast for another 3 hours. Let it cool.

8. Gently remove the brisket from the pocket, without the sauce, and lay the meat on a cutting board. Carve ½" slices, cutting against the grain, I recommend using an electric knife. Transfer to a big baking / serving dish and pour the sauce over it to cover.

9. At this point, you either can serve or freeze the brisket. If you freeze it, take it out of the freezer in the morning, and heat it up an hour before dinner at 300°F.

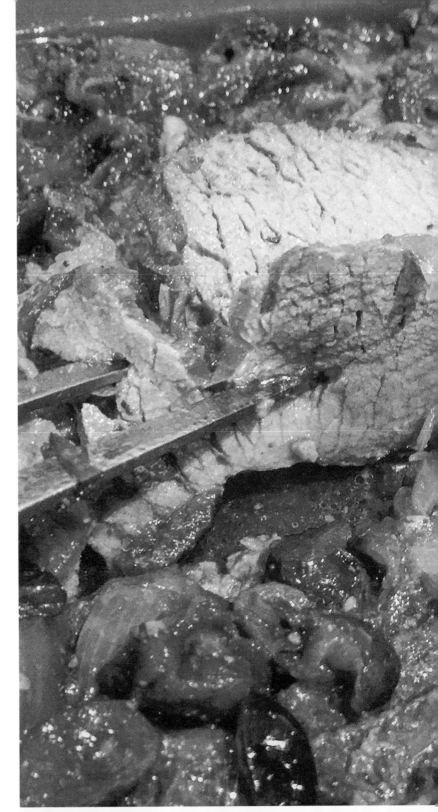

NO LEFTOVERS LAMB SHOULDER

This festive dish is a regular in my kitchen for special holiday meals. It is so easy to make! The key to this recipe is a good piece of meat from a butcher you trust. The butcher will clean the meat, remove any excess fat, and arrange it nicely in a net. Buy the meat the day before you plan to cook, because marinating it overnight gives the best results. The meat comes out so juicy that everyone comes back for seconds—hence the name.

HERE IS WHAT YOU NEED:

4-6 lbs. (approximately) shoulder lamb, cleaned and put in a net

¼ cup olive oil

2-3 rosemary sprigs, chopped coarsely

5 garlic cloves, sliced

½ tablespoon cumin

Salt and pepper

LET'S DO THIS:

1. Prepare the meat by inserting the garlic slices under the netting and in between the meat crevices. Spread the olive oil and spices all over the meat with your hands. Place it in a Ziploc® bag in the refrigerator overnight.

2. When ready to cook, place the lamb in an ovenproof dish and roast at 450°F for 20 minutes, uncovered. Lower the heat to 350°F and continue roasting for a total length of 45 minutes (for a 4-lb. piece) to 1 hour and 15 minutes (for a 6-lb. piece). The lamb is ready when a thermometer placed in the middle of the meat reads 135°F degrees.

3. Remove the meat from the oven, cover it with foil, and let it rest on a cutting board for about 10 minutes. Using scissors, remove the net and slice the meat like a loaf of bread.

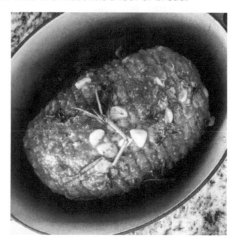

NOT YOUR MOTHER'S MEATLOAF

Short on time? This one is for you! This is actually my Mom's version of meatloaf, which is a bit different from the traditional all-American variety. You can also substitute another kind of ground meat, like chicken or turkey. If you are cooking for two, you can halve the recipe, as this recipe will feed a family of five for two days.

HERE IS WHAT YOU NEED:

2 lbs. ground beef
(high quality, grass-fed)

1 onion, cubed tiny

6 garlic cloves, minced

1 sweet potato, grated

2 eggs, scrambled

1 tablespoon cumin

Salt and pepper

½ bunch parsley, chopped
(optional)

½ cup prepared rice
or quinoa (optional)

1 tablespoon sesame seeds
(to sprinkle on top)

LET'S DO THIS:

1. Combine everything in a big bowl and use your hands to mix well until everything is evenly distributed. Do not over-mix, as this can damage the texture and absorbency of the meat.

2. Grease an oven-safe dish (about 7"x9" in size). Spread the meat evenly and sprinkle sesame seeds all over. Bake at 375°F for 40 minutes.

3. Let cool slightly, cut into 2"x2" size squares, and serve.

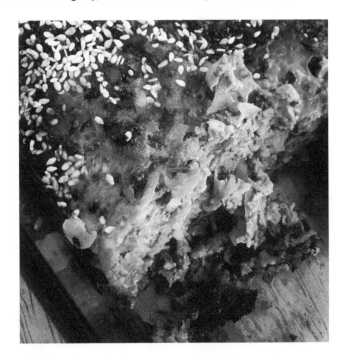

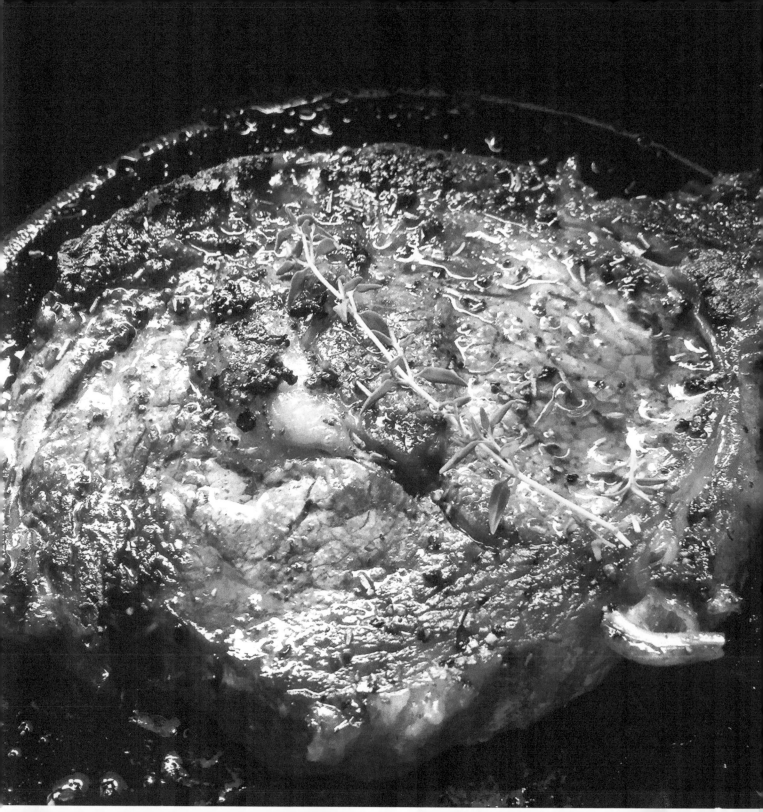

GRILLED SIRLOIN 101

If you love a good cut of beef but are unsure how to prepare it properly, this recipe is for you. Sometimes the most complicated step is to get a high-quality meat, the rest is a piece of pie... I meant steak!

HERE IS WHAT YOU NEED:

1 sirloin steak, patted dry

4 tablespoons olive oil

2 teaspoons cumin

1 teaspoon dried rosemary

1-2 fresh rosemary springs, chopped rough

3 minced garlic cloves (or ½ teaspoons garlic powder)

Salt and black pepper to taste

LET'S DO THIS:

1. Mix all of the ingredients and spread on the sirloin. Place the meat in a Ziploc® bag for a couple of hours or overnight. Press the meat with the heels of your hands, to tenderize.

2. Leave the meat out at room temperature for an hour before grilling. (You can skip this step if you don't have time.)

3. Heat the grill to 400°F. Cook on one side for 10-12 minutes without touching or moving the meat. Flip the meat over and grill for another 10-12 minutes. For medium-well, poke the meat in the center; it should feel firm yet springy. If it feels too bouncy, let it grill for another 5 minutes.

4. Remove the meat from the grill and tent with foil for 5 minutes. Place on a cutting board and slice thinly, cutting against the grain.

FANCY CHUCK ROAST

This hearty dish is perfect for cold weather days to feed a family or guests over the weekend. I have made this recipe ahead of time many times and reheated before serving the day I needed it. The meat tastes even better when reheated, and it still looks beautiful the next day. It might look fancy, but this dish is very simple to make.

HERE IS WHAT YOU NEED:

2-3 lbs. chuck roast

2 tablespoons coconut oil

3 carrots

3 celery stalks

2 onions

5 prunes

5 dried peaches

5 garlic cloves

2 sweet potatoes

2 regular potatoes

2-3 teaspoons sea salt

2 teaspoons black pepper

2 tablespoons cumin

2-3 sprigs of rosemary and sage

2-3 cups vegetable or chicken broth (or water)

Salt and pepper

LET'S DO THIS:

1. Chop all vegetables and dried fruits into large chunks and place in a large stove to oven dish like a Dutch oven. Toss them with 2 tablespoons olive oil and 1 teaspoon of sea salt and the herbs.

2. Prepare the meat by patting it dry, sprinkle with 1 teaspoon sea salt and pepper on both sides. Using a separate large skillet with coconut oil, sauté the roast 5-7 minutes on each side.

3. While the meat is searing on both sides, sauté the vegetable mixture on the stove for about 4-5 minutes on medium heat.

4. Place the seared meat on top of the vegetables and sprinkle generously with salt, pepper, and cumin. Pour the liquids against the sides of the dish and bring to a light boil.

5. Bake at 350°F for 45 minutes, reduce the heat to 250°F and continue baking covered for another two and a half hours.

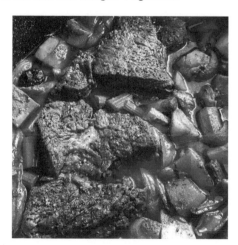

LAMB SHANK

This recipe takes ten minutes of prepare and two hours in the oven, yet produces a gourmet dish that makes everyone lick their fingers and ask for more. It is hearty and very appropriate for the cold-weather months. If you are short on time, prepare the ingredients the day before, then pop in the oven two hours before dinner. I am a big believer that the meat tastes better the day after it has been cooked—so feel free to store the lamb in the fridge and reheat it for a few days after it has been cooked.

HERE IS WHAT YOU NEED:

2 lamb shanks, approximately 3 lbs. each (or other piece of meat bone-in)

6 prunes

2-3 rosemary and thyme sprigs

1 sweet potato, cut into chunks

4 carrots, cut into chunks

2 onion, cut into chunks

1 garlic head (cut in half horizontally)

5-6 celery stalks, cut into chunks

3 tablespoons coconut or olive oil

2 teaspoons turmeric

2 teaspoons garlic powder

Salt and pepper, to taste

2 cups water (or chicken broth)

1 teaspoon cinnamon (optional but adds a lot of flavor!)

LET'S DO THIS:

1. Sprinkle salt and pepper generously all over the meat.

2. In a large stove-to-oven dish, heat the oil and sear the meat for 5 minutes. Turn it over and add the vegetables, prunes, and garlic. Sprinkle everything with the seasonings, while the second side of the meat sears for another 5 minutes. Add the water, herbs and sprinkle on just a bit more sea salt.

3. Cover the dish, transfer to the oven and cook at 300°F for 2 hours.

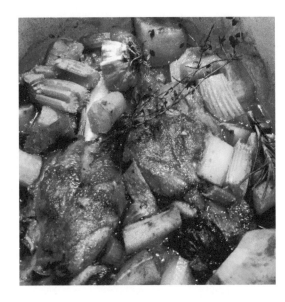

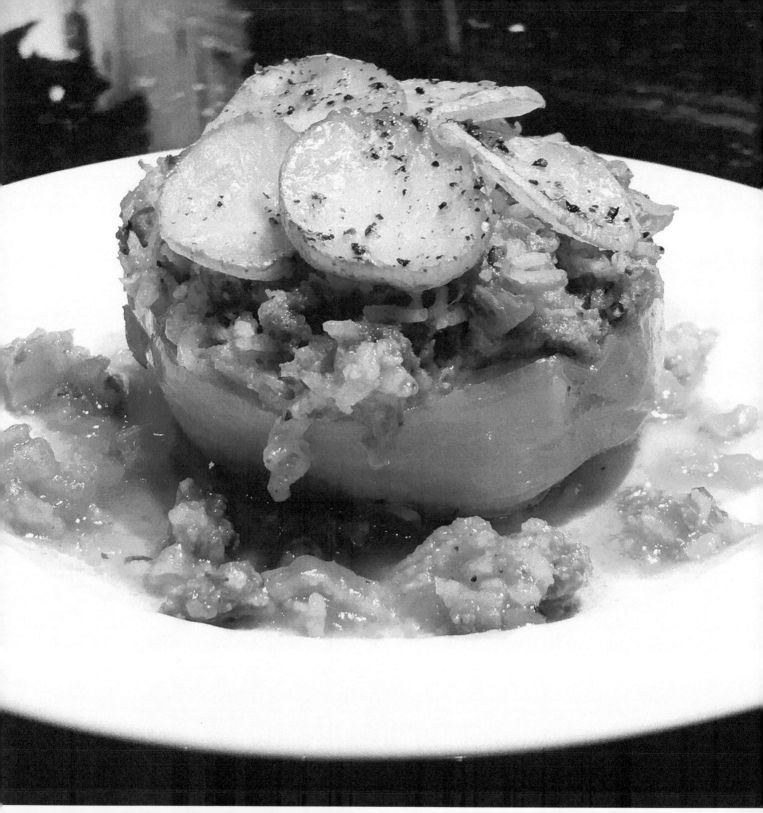

STUFFED RED PEPPERS

———

This delicious recipe is a traditional dish in the Israeli cuisine. You can find it in many versions and combination of spices and vegetables. This version is simple to prepare with wholesome ingredients. To get the most out of your time in the kitchen, double the recipe and freeze a portion for those days you are too busy to cook.

HERE IS WHAT YOU NEED:

3-4 red peppers clean and halved horizontally

Filling:

2 tablespoons olive oil

1 large onion, diced small

1 small fennel, diced small

3 celery stalks, diced small

1 lb. grass fed organic ground beef

1 teaspoon smoked paprika

1 teaspoon garlic powder

1 tablespoon dried oregano

½ cup white basmati rice, rinsed and drained

1 cup water

1 (14.5-ounce) can diced tomatoes

1 (14.5-ounce) can tomato sauce

Salt and pepper

1 fresh tomato or potato, thinly sliced

LET'S DO THIS:

1. Using a large skillet, sauté the onions, celery, and fennel in olive oil until golden.

2. Add the ground beef and sauté until fully cooked. Separate the ground beef using a wooden spoon. Season with salt and pepper.

3. Add to the skillet the cans of tomatoes, rice, water and spices and stir; let it cook on low heat for a few minutes. The rice should not be cooked all the way; it will cook thoroughly later on in the oven. Turn off the heat. If the sauce seems too thick, add a half cup of water.

4. Arrange the peppers open side up in an oven-safe dish and sprinkle with salt and pepper. Fill them up with the meat sauce to their top. Spread the leftover meat sauce all around the peppers.

5. Pour the tomatoe sauce all around the peppers. Top each pepper with thin slices of tomato or potato, brush with olive oil, sprinkle additional oregano, salt, and pepper, and cover the dish with tinfoil.

6. Bake at 350°F for one hour. Uncover and broil for 5 more minutes (this last step is optional)

189

UN-STUFFED CABBAGE

Un-stuffed Cabbage is an easy comfort food and popular dish in my house, especially during the colder months. We love to come home after a long day and enjoy this nourishing dish. Stuffed cabbage reminds me of my grandmother's cooking, but since I don't have the time or patience to follow the traditional recipe, I developed a short cut. Here is the best of both worlds, traditional flavors and an easy preparation. You can serve the cabbage with side of organic basmati rice, but it is equally amazing on its own. It will last for a couple of days in the refrigerator and it freezes well, so you can eat some and save the rest for when you are really, really short on time.

HERE IS WHAT YOU NEED:

1 tablespoon coconut oil

1 onion, cut into thin strips

2 bags shredded cabbage or a small head, shredded

1 (14.5-ounce) can of crushed tomatoes

1 can tomato paste

2 cups water

Juice from 2 lemons

1 handful of dried cranberries

Salt and pepper

Meatballs:

2 lbs. grass-fed ground beef

2 eggs

1 small onion, diced into tiny pieces

Salt and pepper

LET'S DO THIS:

1. In a large pot, heat the oil on medium heat and add the onion. Sauté until light gold. Add the cabbage. Stir and let cook for 5-10 minutes. Add the crushed tomatoes, tomato paste, water, cranberries, salt and pepper, and lemon. Let cook for 10 minutes until it starts boiling. Lower the heat to medium-low.

2. While the sauce is cooking, prepare the meatballs. Thoroughly combine all of the ingredients, roll the mixture into 1" balls, and gently drop them into the bubbling sauce. Use a wooden spoon to distribute the meatballs in the pot.

3. Cover the pot and simmer for 45 minutes on low heat. Taste the sauce and adjust if needed with salt and pepper. Serve warm over quinoa, rice, or cauliflower rice.

4. This recipe stores well in the refrigerator for up to a week.

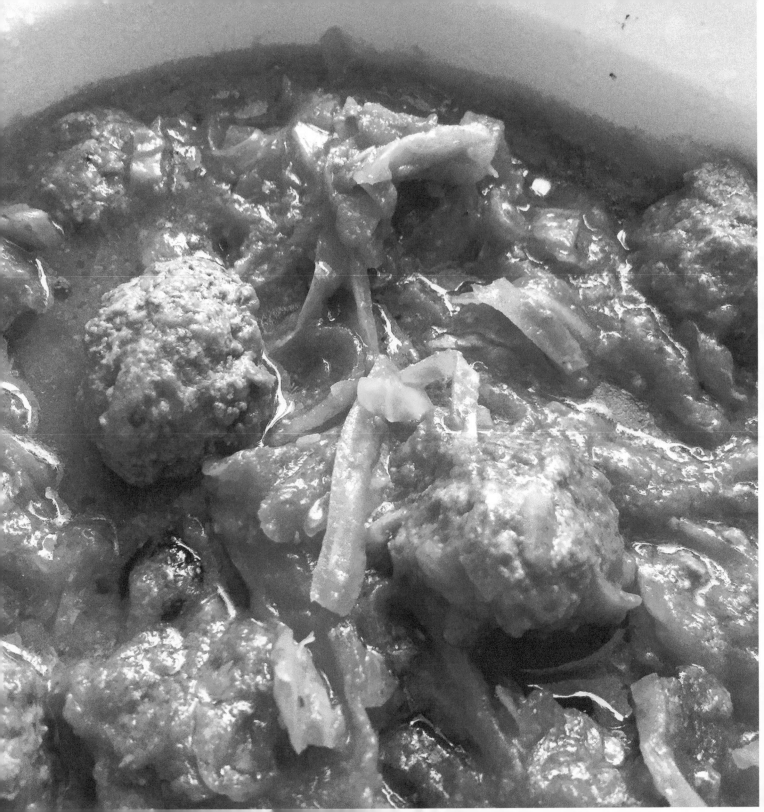

FAVORITE BEEF CUTLETS

Add a few goodies to the beef before cooking, and jazz up an everyday cutlet! You will enjoy new flavors, more nutrients, and meat that is more juicy and tasty. This recipe is one of my family's favorites.

HERE IS WHAT YOU NEED:

1 lb. grass-fed ground beef

1 egg

1 cup chopped sun-dried tomatoes

1 onion, diced small

1 cup parsley, chopped

1-2 garlic cloves, minced

Salt and pepper

1 teaspoon cumin

LET'S DO THIS:

1. In a mixing bowl, combine all of the ingredients using your hands (for better results).

2. Divide the meat into six even portions and shape into patties.

3. You can sauté the cutlets in a skillet on the stove, grill them, or bake on a cookie sheet at 375°F for 30 minutes.

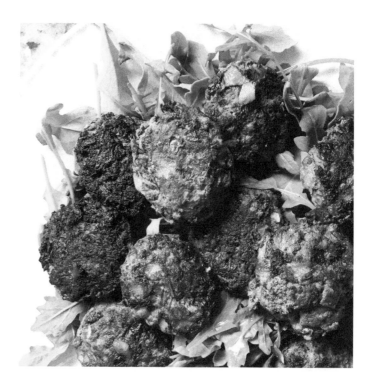

BEEF & CAULIFLOWER HAMBURGERS

Who knew hamburgers could be so healthy? The carnivores in the family won't even realize how many vegetables are hiding in their favorite food. This is a burger you can eat regularly, since it is packed with good-for-you ingredients.

HERE IS WHAT YOU NEED:

1 lb. grass-fed organic ground beef

1 cup shredded cauliflower

2 cups chopped kale or spinach

1 purple onion, chopped small

3 garlic cloves, crushed

¼ cup sun-dried tomatoes, chopped (optional)

2 eggs, scrambled

1 tablespoon cumin

Salt and pepper

2 tablespoons of coconut or olive oil for frying

LET'S DO THIS:

1. Combine all of the ingredients in a large bowl and mix well using your hands. Shape into patties—usually the mixture makes about 6 large or 8 smaller burgers.

2. Lightly coat a pan with oil and set it on medium heat. Fry the cutlets, about 5 minutes on each side.

3. Serve on a bed of baby spinach leaves or use portabella mushrooms or large romaine lettuce leaves as buns.

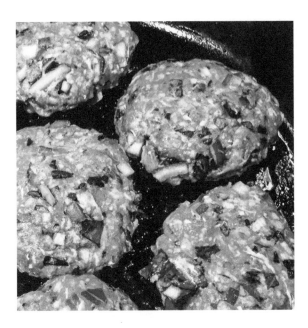

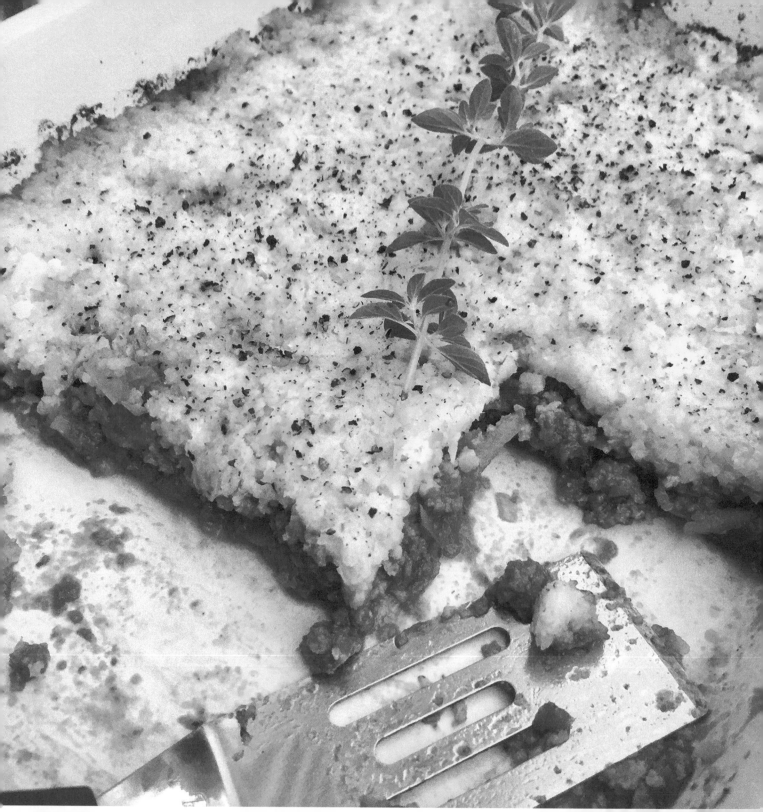

SHEPHERD'S PIE

This is a health-conscious version of an all-American classic dish that is just as filling and tasty as the original. Cauliflower is a high-nutrient veggie that absorbs surrounding flavors beautifully. You can also play with a few variations: substitute the beef with any other ground meat, or make the dish vegetarian by swapping out the meat for 4 cups of finely-chopped mushrooms.

HERE IS WHAT YOU NEED:

Top Layer:

1 head cauliflower broken into medium flowers

1 tablespoon ghee (or butter or coconut oil)

1 tablespoon Dijon mustard

Salt and pepper

Bottom Layer:

2 tablespoons oil

1 onion, diced small

3 carrots, grated

3 stalks celery, diced

1 lbs. grass-fed ground beef (or chicken or turkey)

3 tablespoons tomato paste

1½ cups water

1 egg, scrambled

½ teaspoon mustard powder

Pinch cloves

Pinch cinnamon

Salt and pepper

LET'S DO THIS:

1. In a medium pot, boil the cauliflower in water for 20-25 minutes until soft. Drain and leave in the pot.

2. Add the ghee, mustard, salt, and pepper to the cauliflower. Using a hand-held blender (or potato masher), process the cauliflower with the seasoning until smooth.

3. While the cauliflower is boiling, prepare the bottom layer. Place a large skillet on medium heat; add the oil, and sauté the onions, carrots, celery, and ground beef. Let everything sauté for 10-15 minutes, until the beef is cooked through. Add the tomato paste, water, mustard powder, cloves, cinnamon, and salt and pepper. Continue to cook on low heat until the mixture thickens slightly. Taste and adjust the flavors as needed. Let cool.

4. Add the scrambled egg. Incorporate well with the meat sauce.

5. In an oven-safe dish (like a 9"x13" Pyrex® pan), spread the meat filling evenly, and then spread the cauliflower on top. Sprinkle on a bit more salt and pepper.

6. Bake at 375°F for 30 minutes or until the edges bubble and turn golden brown. Cut into 3"x3" squares and serve.

UPGRADED BEEF BURGERS

This recipe elevates the humble burger by adding leeks (a member of the onion family), which give a rich and delicate flavor to the meat. The optional sesame garnish adds crunch and an earthy, nutty taste that intensifies with cooking. With either addition, these burgers are scrumptious!

HERE IS WHAT YOU NEED:

2 lbs. grass-fed ground beef

2 eggs

Handful of chopped parsley

2 leeks, diced small, boiled to soften, and drained

4 garlic cloves, minced

1 tablespoon cumin

Salt and pepper

Sesame seeds, to garnish (optional)

LET'S DO THIS:

1. Mix all ingredients until well combined and form about 12 medium-size patties. Sprinkle sesame seeds on top and press down lightly, to trap the seeds within the meat.

2. Bake at 375°F for 30-40 minutes. Or sauté in a skillet with 1 tablespoon coconut oil about 4 minutes on each side.

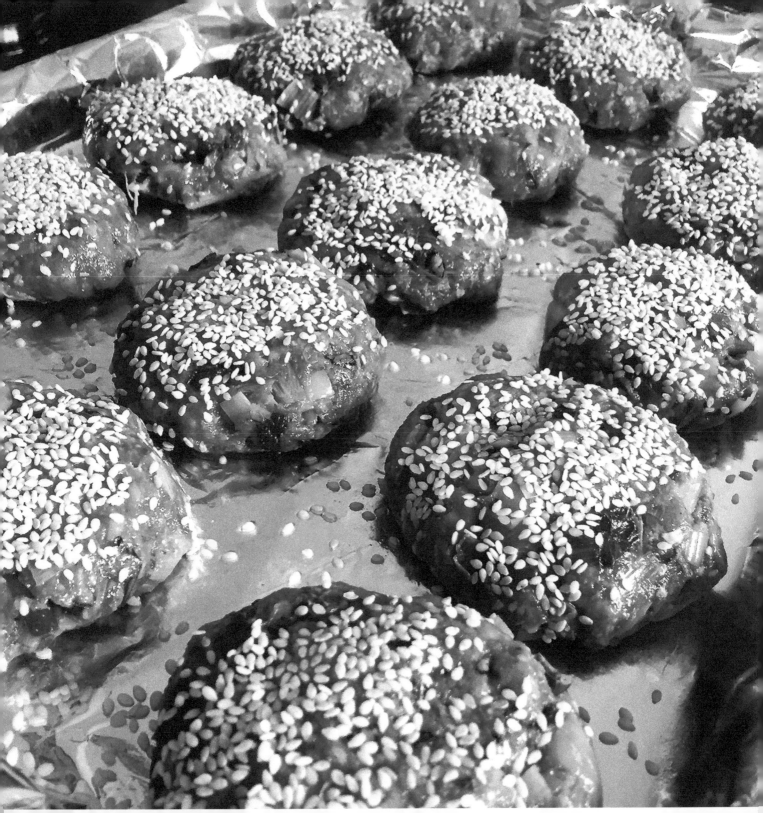

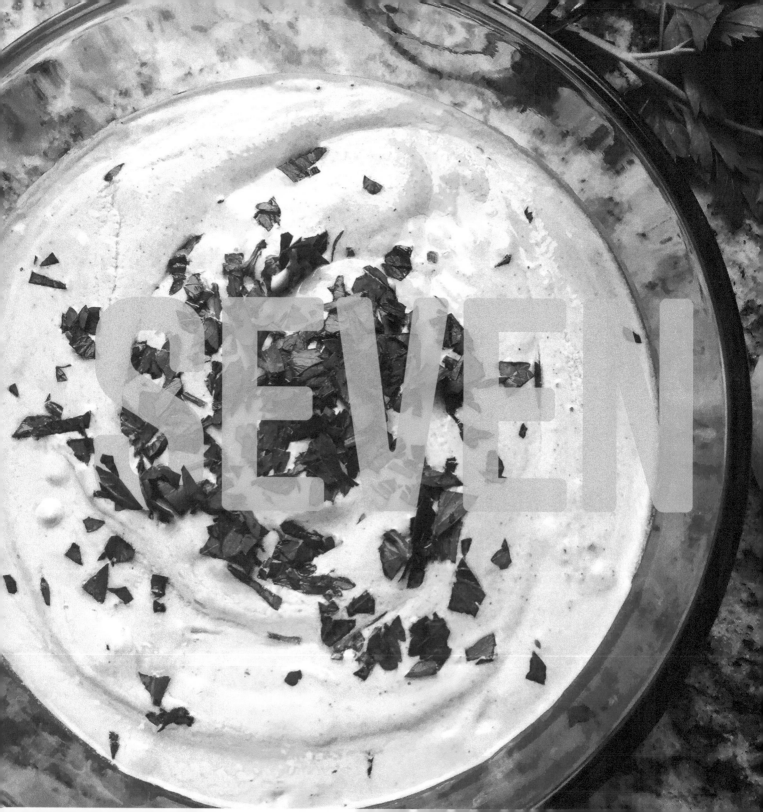

SAUCES
Flavor!

Home made sauces and dips play a big role in my kitchen. Since they take just a few minutes to make, I hope they become a favorite item in your kitchen as well. Sauces can upgrade any simply prepared chicken, fish or veggies, to a gourmet dish. It is always a good idea to double the recipe and use it on different dishes or, alternately, just eat them right out of the jar as a treat!

TAHINI SAUCE

I use tahini a lot in my kitchen, because it adds a rich flavor and is high in protein and other nutrients, including good fats. Raw tahini is a thick paste made from ground sesame seeds, with no flavoring or water added, and is sold today in many food stores. Your supermarket may also stock prepared tahini sauce (often in the refrigerated section), which is the raw paste mixed with water, lemon, garlic and seasonings. Both versions can be used as a salad dressing, dip, or seasoning for roasted vegetables, fish or chicken. It is very easy to prepare tahini sauce at home.

HERE IS WHAT YOU NEED:

1 container raw tahini

Water in room temperature, the same amount as the raw tahini (use the tahini container and fill it up with water)

2 lemons, juice only

4-5 garlic cloves

Salt and pepper

Optional seasonings, use one at a time or all at the same time:

1 cup of parsley, chopped

1 tablespoon cumin

1 teaspoon turmeric

LET'S DO THIS:

1. Combine the ingredients in a food processor or blender until the mixture turns lighter in color and has a smooth texture. If you want a thinner sauce, add another ½ cup of water. Keep in mind, the tahini will thicken once it is chilled in the fridge. Transfer to a glass jar and store in the refrigerator for up to a week.

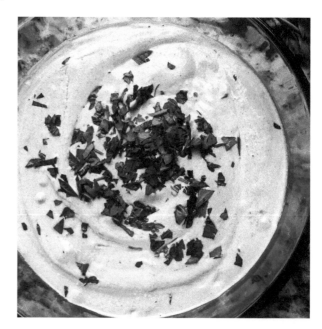

EASY CRANBERRY SAUCE

For years, my mother-in-law was assigned to bring her homemade cranberry sauce for Thanksgiving dinner. I used to devour her sauce by the jar, it was that good! As I gained more knowledge of the ingredients, I decided to develop a healthier version. Don't get me wrong—I love my mother-in-law—but we can always make our traditions healthier. Even she agrees! This delicious recipe contains no refined sugars or chemicals and is very easy to make. I recommend doubling it and enjoying the sauce well beyond Thanksgiving. You can spread it on toast or use it to top your morning oatmeal.

HERE IS WHAT YOU NEED:

8-ounce bag fresh organic cranberries

2 apples, grated

2 carrots, grated

1½ cup water

¼ to ½ cup coconut sugar or maple syrup

Pinch of cinnamon or 1 teaspoon lemond rind

LET'S DO THIS:

1. Combine all of the above in a saucepan and bring to a boil. Lower the heat and cover. Simmer for 20 minutes.

2. Uncover, mix well, and cook on low for another 10-15 minutes.

3. Let the mixture cool and store in the refrigerator up to a week.

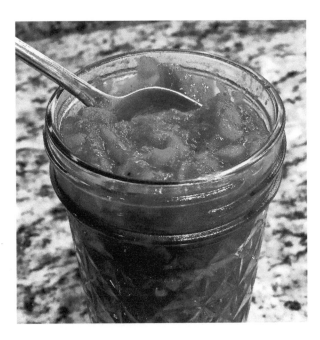

2-MINUTE MAYO

Mayo never tasted as good! Made with simple ingredients, and takes 2 minutes to make, you might not want to use store-bought ever again.

HERE IS WHAT YOU NEED:

1 cup olive oil
1 fresh egg
1 teaspoon Dijon mustard
1 tablespoon lemon juice
Pinch of sea salt

Tall Mason jar
Hand-held blender

LET'S DO THIS:

1. Combine all the ingredients in the jar.

2. Insert the immersion blender into the jar so it touches the bottom. Turn on the blender for about 2 minutes and move it slightly upwards, to make sure everything in the jar is processed.

3. Your mayo is ready! Since it is made from fresh ingredients, be sure to use it within a week.

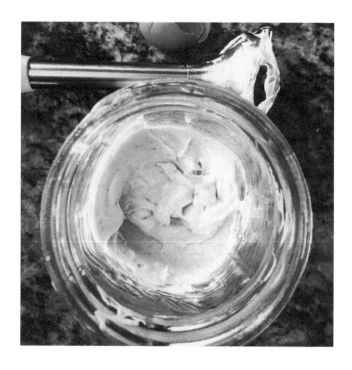

PARSLEY AIOLI

Add a spoonful of this aioli on top of simply prepared fish or chicken, use it as a vegetable dip, or as a salad dressing. It is that versatile!

HERE IS WHAT YOU NEED:

¼ cup olive oil

1 cup parsley

2 garlic cloves, chopped

Salt and pepper

Juice from 1 lemon

LET'S DO THIS:

1. Combine all the ingredients in a tall jar and process using a hand-held blender (or a food processor) until a smooth paste is formed.

2. Refrigerate and use within one week.

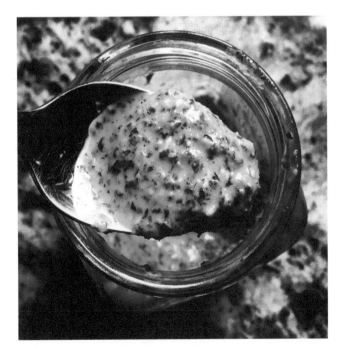

Seeds for Thought... Fat is good for you! Here are some good sources of fat: avocado, avocado oil, coconut oil, olive oil, nuts and seeds, grass-fed butter.

SPICE IT UP AND MAKE IT YOUR OWN

Spices and herbs not only make our food more appetizing and aromatic, but they also deliver loads of health benefits as well. For example, turmeric has anti-inflammatory properties and can be added to both dishes and drinks to boost our immune system. Every cuisine on the globe has its distinctive combination of seasoning, and we can all learn from one another. Explore any of the spices below and bring new tastes into your marinades, coatings, or side dishes. You can sprinkle these seasonings on fish or chicken, or blend them with olive oil to create a marinade. Seasoning with spices can be intimidating at first, but with some practice and the guide below, you will be cooking exotic dishes in no time. Bellow, you will find a simple guide to various spice blends representing different cuisines. Use it as an inspiration and invitation to explore and create new flavors in your kitchen. Don't forget always to add sea salt and freshly ground pepper for taste. Let's see, what cuisine do you want to explore today?

MIDDLE EASTERN / MEDITERRANEAN:

Cilantro, Cumin, Garlic (fresh or powdered), Lemon, Olive oil, Paprika, Parsley, Rosemary, Sumac, Za'atar

SPANISH:

Cayenne pepper, Garlic, Olive oil, Oregano, Paprika, Parsley, Rosemary, Saffron

ASIAN:

Coconut aminos (or soy sauce), Ginger (fresh or powdered), Sesame oil, Sesame seeds, Sugar (coconut sugar)

THE GRILL (BBQ, SEARING):

Garlic, Ground chili peppers, Onion, Oregano, Paprika, Peppercorns, Rosemary, Thyme

INDIAN:

Cardamom, Cinnamon, Cloves, Coriander, Cumin, Curry, Saffron, Turmeric

ITALIAN:

Basil, Capers, Chili peppers, Olive oil, Oregano, Rosemary, Thyme, Tomato sauce

JAMAICAN:

Allspice, Chili pepper, Cinnamon, Dried oregano, Garlic powder, Ground ginger, Lime juice, Nutmeg, Onion powder, Salt and pepper, Sugar (coconut sugar), Thyme, Vinegar

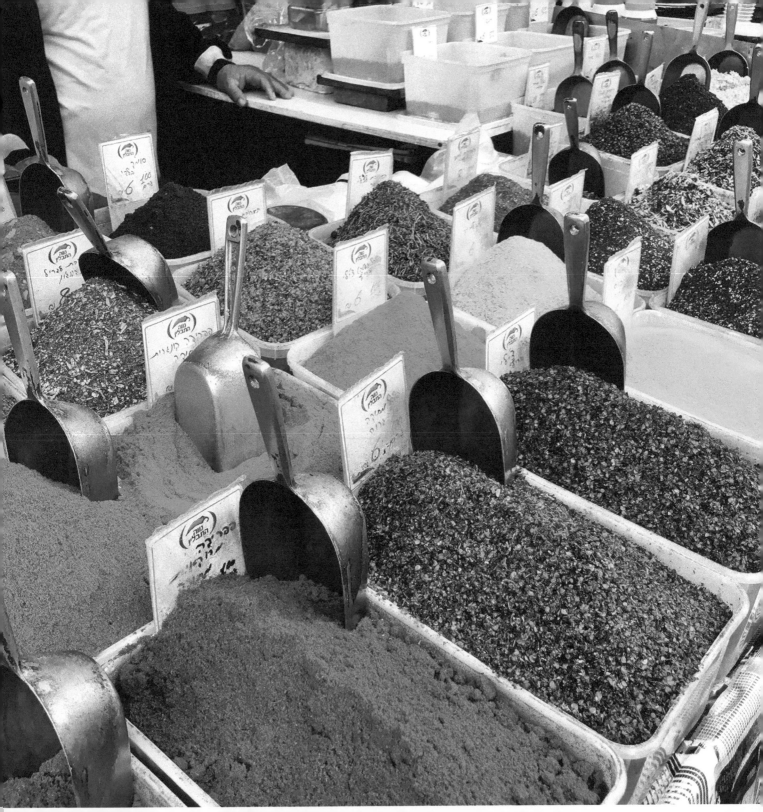

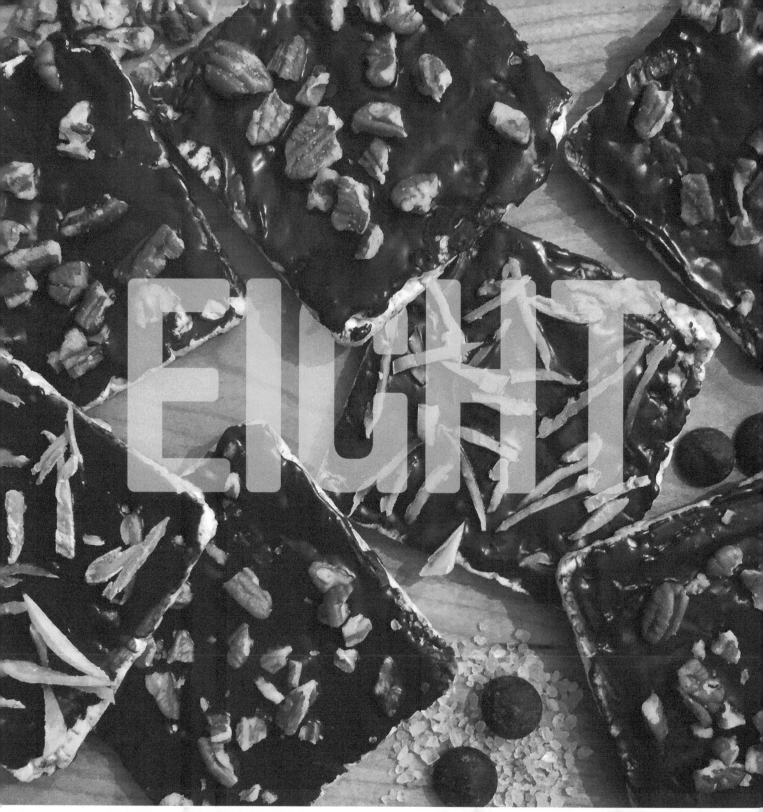

DESSERTS
No Guilt!

This section is full of tasty desserts using whole foods only. The main ingredients in this section include almond meal, coconut sugar, and eggs, all with a high nutritional value that you can enjoy without feeling guilty.

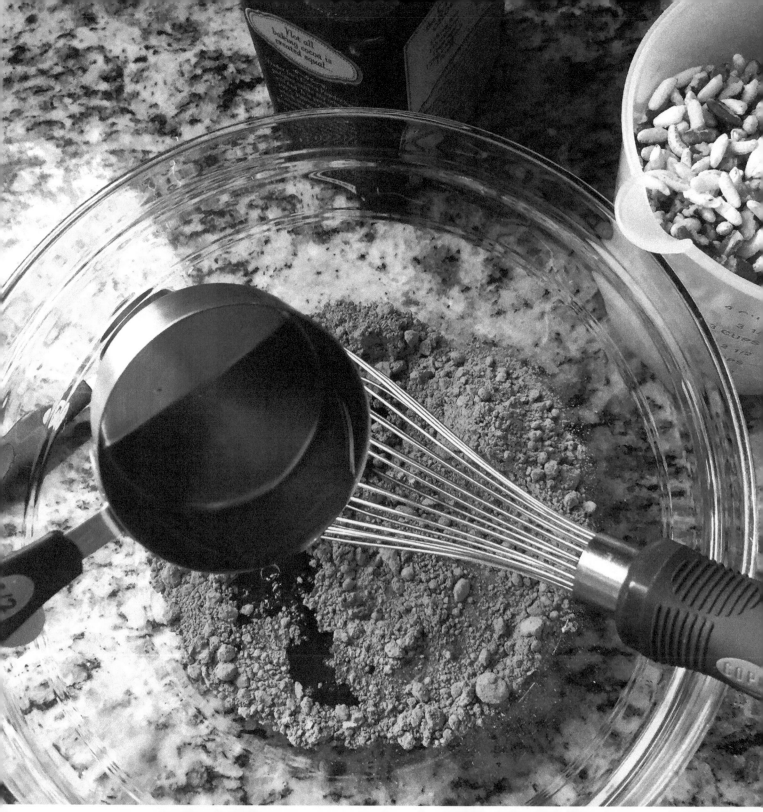

BAKING ESSENTIALS

———

Here is a list of staples to stock up on in the kitchen, so you are always ready to make one of these easy and healthy desserts. I like to keep all of my baking essentials in two plastic containers in the pantry so I can place them on the counter when I am ready to bake. It saves time and keep you organized when the recipe calls for many ingredients.

BAKING STAPLES:
Choose organic whenever available
Eggs
Almond flour
Coconut flour
Arrowroot flour
Cocoa powder (unsweetened)
Flaxseeds meal
Shredded coconut
Baking soda
Baking powder
Coconut sugar
Maple syrup
Grass fed butter
Coconut oil
Olive oil
Sea salt
Chocolate Chips (preferred with high content of cocoa)
Bananas
Apples
Frozen berries
Pecans, almonds
Cinnamon

TOOLS AND EQUIPMENT:
Mixer (free-standing or hand-held)
Food processor
High Power Blender
Spatulas
Wisk
Mixing bowls
Cookie sheets lined with slip mat or parchment paper
Oven safe ceramic dishes
Muffin pans
Cooling rack
Round cake pan
Pie dishes
Cast iron skillet

HEAVENLY COCONUT MACAROONS

This version of the all-time favorite coconut macaroons is simple to make and contains only unrefined and wholesome ingredients. It is a great example of a scrumptious dessert that is actually oh-so-good-for-you! Pack for lunch or eat for breakfast and enjoy the health benefits of coconut, eggs and coconut sugar.

TO GET READY:

Cookie sheet lined with non-stick baking mat or parchment paper

Mixer

Heat the oven to 350°F

HERE IS WHAT YOU NEED:

4 eggs

Pinch salt

4 cups unsweetened coconut flakes, thinly shredded

4 tablespoons coconut sugar

3 tablespoons maple syrup

Chocolate drizzle:

½ cup chocolate chips

1 tablespoon butter or coconut oil

LET'S DO THIS:

1. Place the eggs in a mixer bowl. Begin mixing on slow speed, then gradually raise the speed to high. Add a pinch of salt and continue to mix on high. Start adding the sugar, one tablespoon at a time. Do the same with the maple syrup.

2. Add another pinch of salt and continue mixing on high for another 5 minutes, until the egg mixture develops light, fluffy, golden folds. Turn off the mixer and put the bowl on the counter.

3. With a large spatula and gentle folding motions, add the coconut to the beaten eggs, one cup at a time, until everything is combined.

4. Using a tablespoon, scoop the batter into rounded domes on a cookie sheet lined with a non-stick baking mat or parchment paper. Bake at 350°F for 20-25 minutes or until the edges of the macaroons are golden brown.

5. While the macaroons cool, prepare the chocolate drizzle by melting the chocolate chips and oil in a small saucepan on low heat. Drizzle the sauce over the macaroons and let cool before serving.

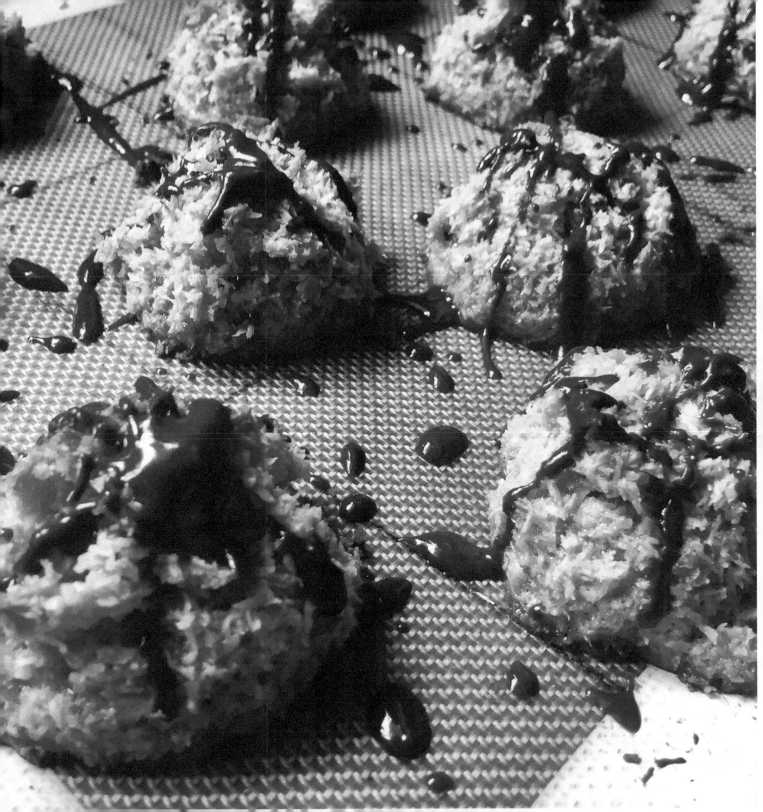

CINNAMON MUFFINS

These cinnamon muffins are so simple to make and no one will suspect they are good for you!

TO GET READY:

Muffin pan

Parchment cupcake liners

Mixer

Heat the oven to 350°F

HERE IS WHAT YOU NEED:

4 eggs

⅓ cup coconut sugar

¼ cup coconut oil

1 teaspoon vanilla

Pinch salt

1½ cups almond flour

¼ cup coconut flour

2 tablespoons arrowroot flour

¼ teaspoon baking powder

¼ teaspoon baking soda

¼ teaspoon cinnamon

Cinnamon topping:

3 tablespoons maple syrup

2 tablespoons coconut sugar

1 tablespoon almond meal

2 tablespoon coconut oil (melted)

¼ teaspoon cinnamon

LET'S DO THIS:

1. Using a mixer on medium speed, begin by mixing the eggs and sugar. Slowly add the oil, then the vanilla and salt.

2. Pause the mixer and add the dry ingredients. Mix well. Scoop the batter into the muffin liners, leaving ¾ " of space from the top of each muffin.

3. In a separate bowl, mix together the topping ingredients with a small spoon. Drizzle a spoonful on top of each muffin and briefly swirl it into the batter; don't blend it completely. Bake at 350°F for 20 minutes or until the edges of the muffins turn golden brown. Let the muffins cool for 5 minutes in the pan, then transfer them to a cooling rack.

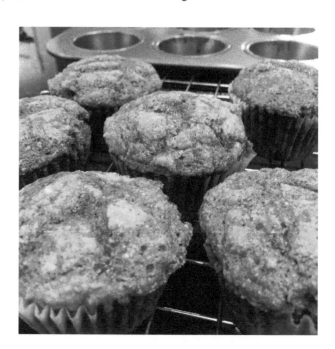

CHOCOLATE COCONUT BALLS

These treats are truly addictive—but not to worry, they are packed with wholesome nutrients that your body can use as fuel. Think of them as round, tiny power bars.

TO GET READY:

Food processor

HERE IS WHAT YOU NEED:

2 cups pitted dates, soaked in water for a half hour and drained

½ cup almond meal

⅓ cup cocoa powder

½ cup toasted almond or pecan

½ cup shredded coconut

2 tablespoons flaxseed meal

½ teaspoon grated lemon rind

Pinch of sea salt

For Garnish: Sesame seeds, cocoa powder, shredded coconut, or goji berries

LET'S DO THIS:

1. Combine everything in a food processor until all becomes a thick paste. If the mixture is too dry, add 2-3 tablespoon water. If the mixture is too wet, add a little more shredded coconut and process again.

2. Create 1" balls. Roll them in coating of your choice. Simply place the garnish in a small bowl and roll the chocolate balls in it. Store the balls in an airtight container in the freezer or the refrigerator. They will keep fresh in the freezer up to a month and in the refrigerator up to two weeks.

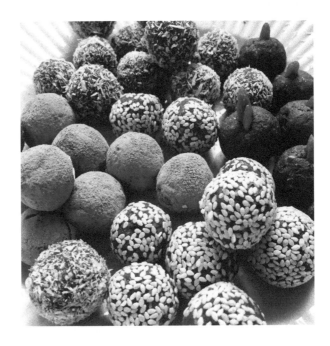

VERY FUDGY BROWNIES

If you like your brownies dense, fudgy, and extra chocolaty, this recipe is for you! In the same amount of time it takes to use a boxed mix, you will have something far more scrumptious.

TO GET READY:

Mixer

8"x8" square glass dish

Heat the oven to 350°F

HERE IS WHAT YOU NEED:

½ cup soft butter
   or coconut oil

1 cup coconut sugar

2 eggs

⅓ cup unsweetened
   cocoa powder

¾ cup almond flour/meal

2 heaping tablespoons
   arrowroot flour or
   potato starch

Pinch teaspoon salt

½ cup chocolate chips

Extra chocolate chips to
   sprinkle on top just before
   baking (optional)

LET'S DO THIS:

1. Place butter / oil, sugar, and eggs in a mixer bowl. Mix very well on low speed, then gradually increase the speed to medium-high speed. Mix for 4-5 minutes.

2. Pause the mixer, add the rest of the ingredients, then mix well on low speed until the batter is thick and even.

3. Stop the mixer, scrape the ingredients from the bottom of the bowl, and resume mixing on medium speed for 3 minutes.

4. In the meantime, melt the chocolate chips.

5. Pause the mixer again, then add the melted chocolate chips and continue mixing until everything is combined.

6. Transfer to a greased, glass, oven-safe dish and bake at 350°F for 20 minutes. The brownies are ready when the edges start to separate from the dish. Let them cool for half hour before serving.

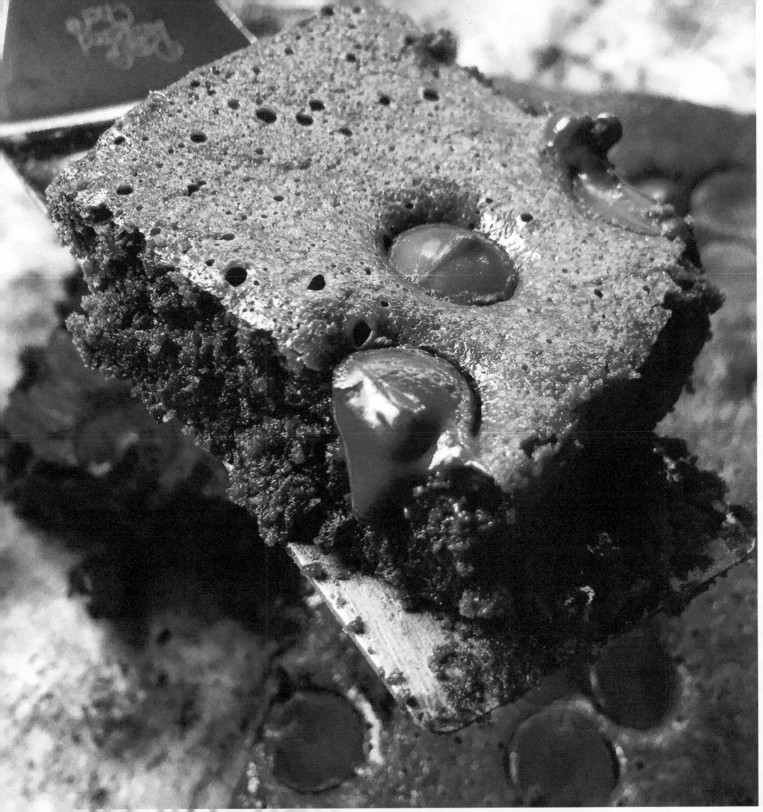

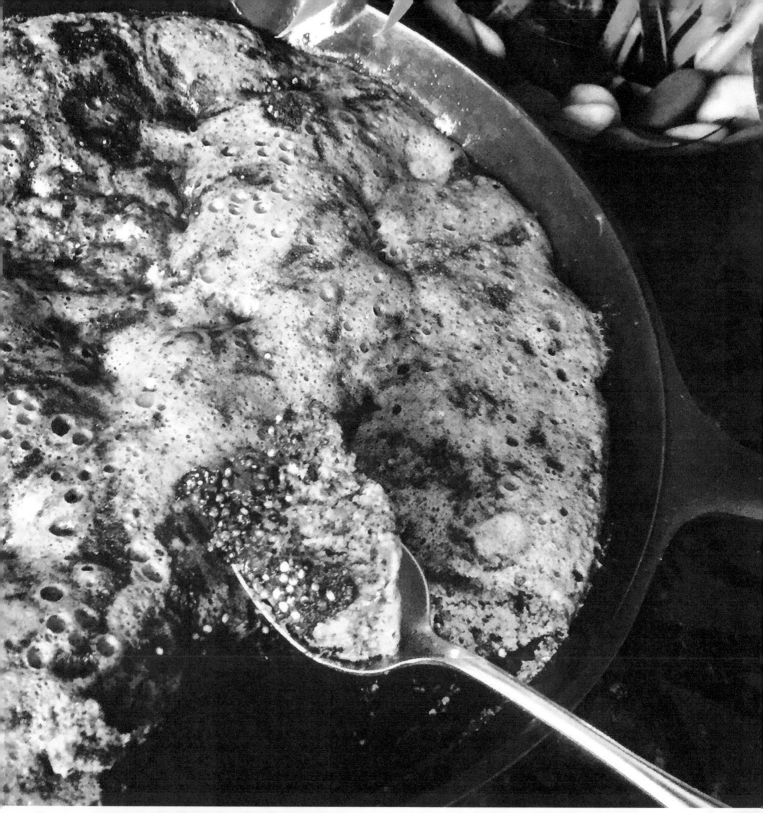

RUSTIC BLUEBERRY COBBLER

This bright, simple cake can be done in a cast-iron skillet or an oven-safe glass/ceramic dish, your choice! The quinoa adds body to the blueberries and a powerhouse of nutrients. Serve on it's own or with a scoop of vanilla ice cream on top.

TO GET READY:

Cast iron skillet or any skillet

or

Round pie dish

Mixing bowl

Heat the oven to 350°F

HERE IS WHAT YOU NEED:

Blueberry mixture:

1 bag frozen blueberries
  (2 cups)

1 tablespoon coconut oil

¼ cup dry quinoa

Batter:

1 cup almond meal

3 eggs

¼ cup coconut sugar

¼ cup olive oil or coconut oil

¼ teaspoon baking soda

¼ teaspoon baking powder

Sprinkle of cinnamon
  (optional)

LET'S DO THIS:

1. Using a 9" cast-iron skillet, heat the oil and add the blueberries. When the blueberries start to bubble, add the quinoa and keep cooking on low heat for about 5 minutes.

2. In the meantime, use a separate bowl to mix the batter ingredients with a fork or whisk.

3. For the cast-iron version: Pour the batter over the blueberries and swirl them together gently with a wooden spoon. Transfer the cast-iron pan to the oven and bake at 350°F for 20 minutes.

4. For the pie plate version: Once the blueberries and the batter are ready, pour the blueberries into a greased pie dish. Add the batter on top and swirl gently with a spoon, until some of the blueberries are at the top of the mixture. Bake at 350°F for 30 minutes.

SUMMER PEACH COBBLER

Need a dessert but short on time? This is a great recipe that takes only a few minutes to prepare. It is refreshing and packed with healthy ingredients. You can use a cast-iron skillet or a ceramic pie dish. Either way, it will be delicious!

TO GET READY:

Cast iron skillet

or

Round Pie dish

Mixing bowl

Heat the oven to 350°F

HERE IS WHAT YOU NEED:

Peach mixture:

6 peaches, cored and sliced into wedges

1 tablespoon coconut oil or butter

Batter:

3 eggs

1 cup almond meal

3 tablespoons olive oil or melted butter

¼ teaspoon baking soda

¼ cup coconut sugar

Dash cinnamon (optional)

LET'S DO THIS:

1. Heat a cast-iron skillet (if you don't have cast iron, use another pan) on medium. Add the coconut oil and peaches. Cook for 4-5 minutes, or until they soften a little and their juices start to bubble.

2. In a separate bowl, combine all of the batter ingredients.

3. If you are using a cast-iron skillet, add the batter to the peaches in the skillet and swirl them together gently, not too much. Continue cooking on the stove for a few more minutes, then transfer to the oven and bake at 350°F for 20 minutes.

4. If you are using a ceramic dish for baking, pour the peaches into the dish and add the batter on top. Using a spoon, lightly swirl the batter into the peaches. Try to bring a few peaches to the top of the mixture. Bake at 350°F for 35 minutes, or until the edges of the cobbler turn a golden color.

5. Let cool for 30 minutes. Serve at room temperature or while the cobbler is still slightly warm.

Optional: Serve with ice cream on top for a classic American taste.

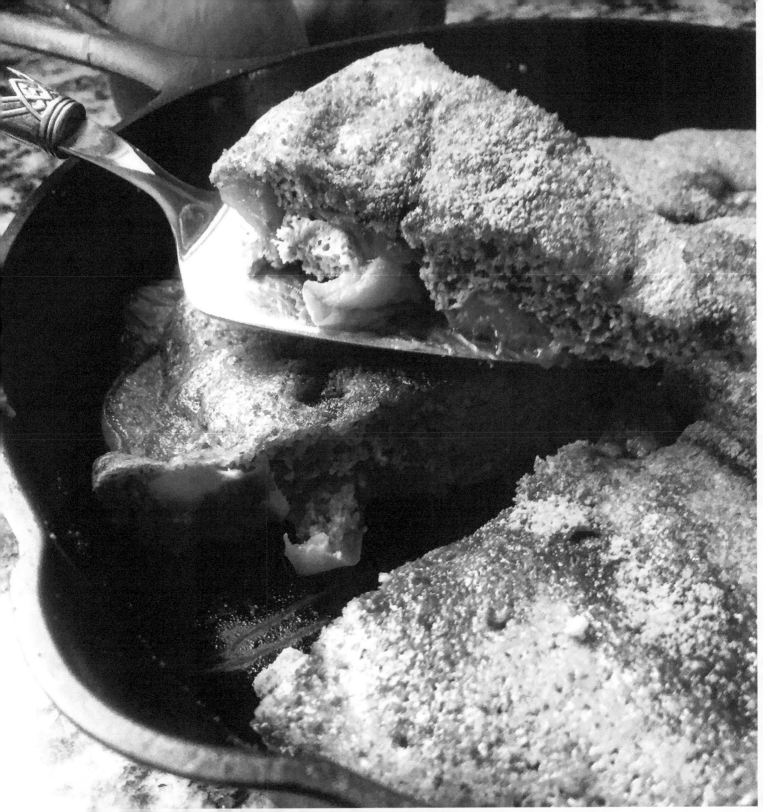

DOUBLE CHOCOLATE CUPCAKES

Love chocolate? This one is for you! They will keep fresh for a few days and they are perfect to send in a lunch box or keep at home as a snack because they are made of good-for-you ingredients.

TO GET READY:

Muffin pan lined with 12 liners

Mixer

Heat the oven to 350°F

HERE IS WHAT YOU NEED:

4 eggs

¾ cup coconut sugar (or 1 cup if you like them sweeter)

¼ cup melted coconut oil

1 teaspoon vanilla

Pinch of salt

1 cup almond meal

⅓ cup unsweetened cocoa powder

1 heaping tablespoon arrowroot flour

¼ teaspoon baking soda

¼ teaspoon baking powder

¾ cup chocolate chips

¼ cup chocolate chips for garnish before baking (optional)

LET'S DO THIS:

1. In a mixer bowl, beat the eggs on medium speed. Continue adding the rest of the ingredients in the order they appear, making sure each is well-incorporated. Lastly, add the chocolate chips and mix well.

2. Scoop the batter into the cups and fill only ¾ of the way up. Garnish with a few chocolate chips on top on each cupcake.

3. Bake at 350°F for 20 minutes and let them cool on a cooling rack.

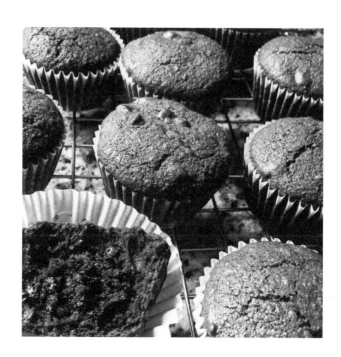

APPLE BERRY CRUMBLE

This is a great dessert after a heavy meal because it is fruity and light, and most of all it is healthy for you! This crumble usually doesn't last more than a day in our home, as it is a real favorite. You can add some sweetness to the bottom fruit layer by adding 2 tablespoons of either maple syrup or coconut sugar, but the baked apples and berries are plenty sweet on their own. Serve this crumble warm or at room temperature, with or without full-fat whipped cream or high quality ice cream.

TO GET READY:

Round ceramic or glass pie dish

Heat the oven on 350°F

HERE IS WHAT YOU NEED:

5 apples (any kind) peeled, cored and chopped into small pieces

1–2 cups frozen berries (blueberries, raspberries, or mixed

Crumble:

½ cup oats

½ cup almond meal

½ cup coconut sugar

¼ cup melted butter (or melted coconut oil)

Handful chopped pecan pieces

Optional: Sprinkle of cinnamon

LET'S DO THIS:

1. Fill a glass / ceramic round pie dish with the apples and berries.

2. In a separate medium-size bowl, combine the crumble ingredients and mix well.

3. Pour the crumble mixture over the fruit. Spread evenly and bake at 350°F for 45 minutes or until the crumble is nice and brown.

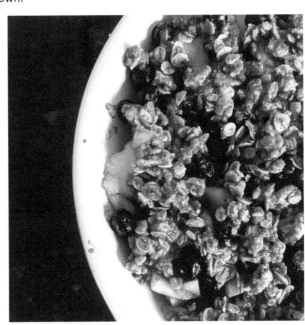

VERY BLUEBERRY MUFFINS

This is a quick and easy recipe that leads to a delicious and nutritious treat. It is packed with antioxidants and can be a great snack to keep around the kitchen. I would recommend storing them in the refrigerator, to make sure the blueberries stay fresh longer.

TO GET READY:

Line a muffin pan with
  12 paper cups

Mixer

Heat the oven to 350°F

HERE IS WHAT YOU NEED:

4 eggs

¾ cup coconut sugar

¼ cup coconut oil (or olive oil)

¼ teaspoon lemon rind

1½ cups almond flour

½ cup arrowroot flour
  (or potato starch)

2 tablespoons coconut flour

¼ teaspoon baking powder

2 cups fresh or frozen wild
  blueberries (set aside a ½ cup
  to use as a garnish)

LET'S DO THIS:

1. In a mixer bowl, combine all the ingredients starting with the eggs and slowly adding the rest in the order they appear. Do not add the blueberries yet. Mix for about 3 minutes until well combined. Turn off the mixer and place the bowl on the counter.

2. Fold in the blueberries, just enough to distribute them evenly.

3. Scoop the batter into the paper cups, leaving ¼" of space from the top. Garnish with a few blueberries on top.

4. Bake at 350°F for 30 minutes. Let cool on a cooling rack.

Seeds for Thought... *Use parchment paper baking cups, or liners, when baking muffins or cupcakes. They make cleanup easy, are non-stick, and they are safe for your health.*

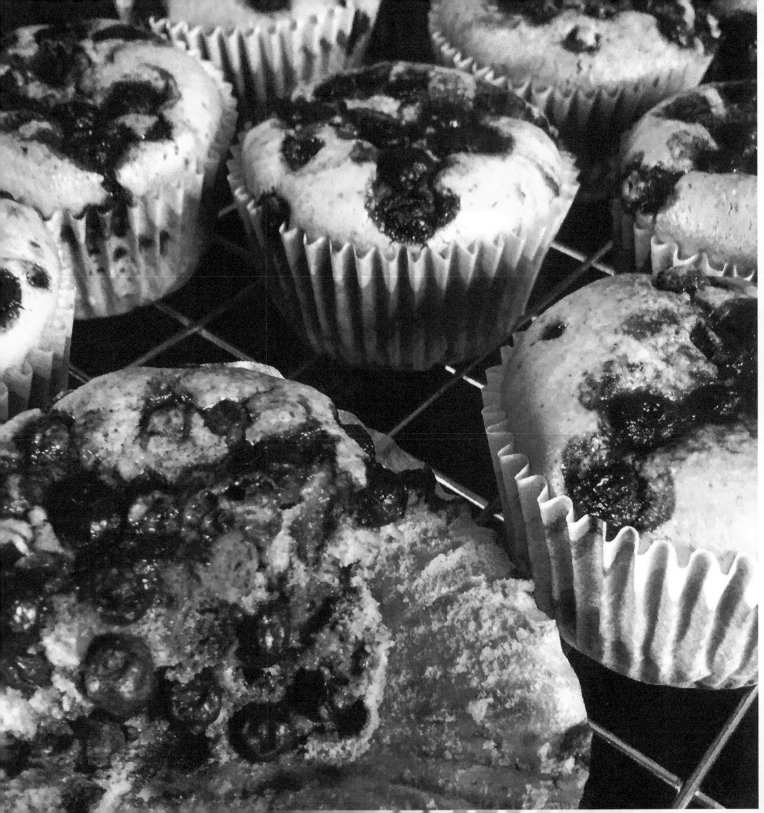

BUTTERNUT SQUASH SQUARES

Don't be fooled by the name—when you serve these squares, no one will know they contain butternut squash and other wholesome ingredients. Once baked, the squash releases a rich, sweet flavor that is a game changer. You can double the maple syrup or sugar, for even sweeter, more crowd-pleasing squares.

TO GET READY:

9"x13" rectangular baking pan lined with parchment paper

Blender

Heat the oven on 350°F

HERE IS WHAT YOU NEED:

1 ½ cups roasted pumpkin or butternut squash (canned organic pumpkin works as well)

⅓ cup coconut sugar or maple syrup

6 eggs

½ cup coconut oil

Dash cinnamon

¾ cup coconut flour

¾ cup almond meal

¼ cup arrowroot flour

1 teaspoon baking soda

1 cup chocolate chips

LET'S DO THIS:

1. In a food processor or blender bowl, mix together all the ingredients except the chocolate chunks / chips, just until blended.

2. Add the chocolate chips and mix well using a flexible spatula.

3. Spread the mixture in a 9"x13" pan lined with parchment paper and bake at 350°F for 30 minutes.

4. Let cool and cut into squares.

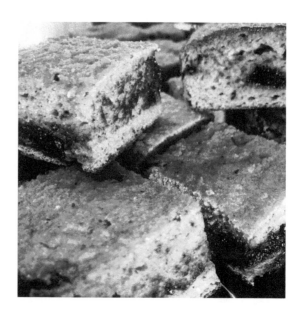

CHOCOLATE RICE CRISPIES

Light and crispy, this dessert is not only fun to eat but fun to make! It is low in sugar, contains antioxidants from the cocoa powder, and good fat from the coconut oil. What more can we want?

TO GET READY:

Large mixing bowl

Muffin pan lined with 12 paper cups

HERE IS WHAT YOU NEED:

2 ½ cups puffed rice (unsweetened and organic)

Chocolate Sauce:

6 tablespoons unsweetened cocoa powder

4 tablespoons maple syrup

½ cup melted coconut oil (or butter)

Pinch salt

LET'S DO THIS:

1. Use a large mixing bowl to combine the cocoa powder, maple syrup, salt, and melted coconut oil. Mix until smooth.

2. Add the puffed rice to the chocolate sauce. Using a spatula, fold together in sweeping motions until the puffs are completely coated with chocolate.

3. Scoop the mix into the muffin cups with a tablespoon. Place in the refrigerator for an hour or more to firm.

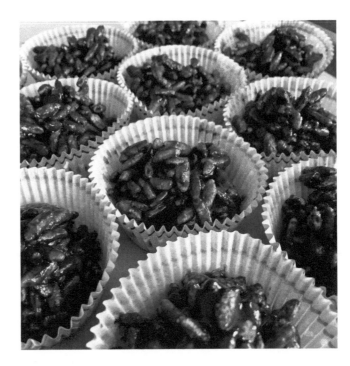

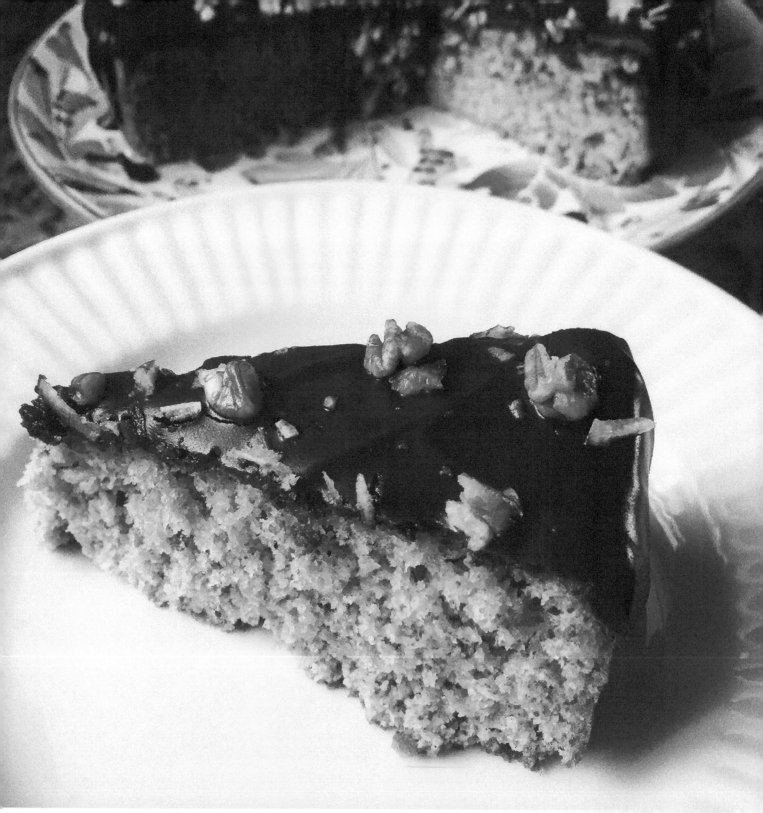

CHOCOLATE COVERED TORTE

A torte is a simple and light cake that can be dressed with any frosting or topping such as fruit or whipped cream. Here is a recipe for a chocolate covered torte that can be found regularly in my Mom's kitchen. I converted the traditional recipe, which included white flour, to a healthier version that contains no white flour or refined sugar.

TO GET READY:
Heat the oven to 350°F
Round springform pan
Mixer
Mixing bowl
2 small sauce pans

HERE IS WHAT YOU NEED:
6 large eggs
10 tablespoon coconut sugar
Pinch of salt
1 ½ cups almond meal
⅓ cup arrowroot flour
½ teaspoon baking powder
½ cup thinly shredded,
    unsweetened coconut
¼ cup small pecan pieces

Syrup:
1 cup water
1 tablespoon vanilla extract
2 tablespoons maple syrup

Frosting:
1 cup chocolate chips
4 tablespoons butter
2 tablespoons milk
    (almond or rice milk is ok)

Garnish:
2 tablespoons chopped
    pecans or walnuts for garnish
2 tablespoons shredded
    coconut for garnish

LET'S DO THIS:

1. Break the eggs into a mixer bowl. Begin mixing at low speed, then gradually increase to high speed. While mixing, add the salt and sugar slowly, one tablespoon at a time. Continue mixing on high for another 12-15 minutes, until the mixture is light and fluffy.

2. While the eggs are beating, mix the dry ingredients together in a separate bowl.

3. Set the two bowls next to each other. With a wide spatula, fold the dry ingredients gradually into the egg mixture. Stir in large, folding movements, being careful not to "break" the fluffy eggs mixture, until just combined.

4. Pour gently into the springform pan. Bake at 350°F for 30 minutes or until the cake begins to separate from the sides of the pan.

5. Set the cake on the counter to cool. It can be frosted in the pan, or you can remove it carefully from the pan in order to frost the sides.

6. Combine the water, vanilla and maple syrup in a small saucepan and bring them to a gentle boil on the stove. Let simmer for 5 minutes. Pour the hot syrup over the cooling cake, then let the cake cool completely.

7. Using a small saucepan on very low heat, melt the chocolate chips with the milk and butter until the mixture is shiny and smooth. Pour over the cake and garnish with shredded coconut, chopped walnuts, or pecans. Let cool completely.

8. Store covered in the refrigerator up to five days.

NO-BAKE CHOCOLATE BANANA CAKE

If the combination of chocolate and bananas gets your attention, this cake is for you! This unusual cake is made with healthy ingredients and has no baking involved. The top and bottom layers are chocolate flavored and the middle layers resembles banana pudding flavor. It is best to keep it in the freezer and take out just half hour before serving.

TO GET READY:
Blender or food processor
Round glass pie dish
Sauce pan

HERE IS WHAT YOU NEED:
Bottom Layer:
10-oz dates, pitted
½ cup almonds
½ cup shredded coconut
2 tablespoon cocoa powder

Middle Layer:
2 bananas
1-cup cashews (soaked overnight in water and drained)
1 can pre-refrigerated coconut milk (just the paste, save the liquid for the top layer)
3 heaping tablespoons rice flour or coconut flour
1 teaspoon vanilla extract
1 tablespoon maple syrup

Top Layer:
¾ cup chocolate chips
¼ cup coconut milk (from the middle layer)
1 banana for garnish

LET'S DO THIS:

1. For the bottom layer, blend all ingredients together in a food processor until well-combined and just a little coarse. Spread tightly in a round pie dish. Place in the freezer for 20-30 minutes.

2. For the middle layer, blend all of the ingredients together on high power in blender until very smooth. Pour over the crust. Freeze for 20-30 minutes.

3. For the top layer, combine both ingredients in a saucepan and melt over very low heat until smooth. Pour over the banana filling. Refrigerate for 4-5 hours or overnight before serving.

4. Garnish with banana slices.

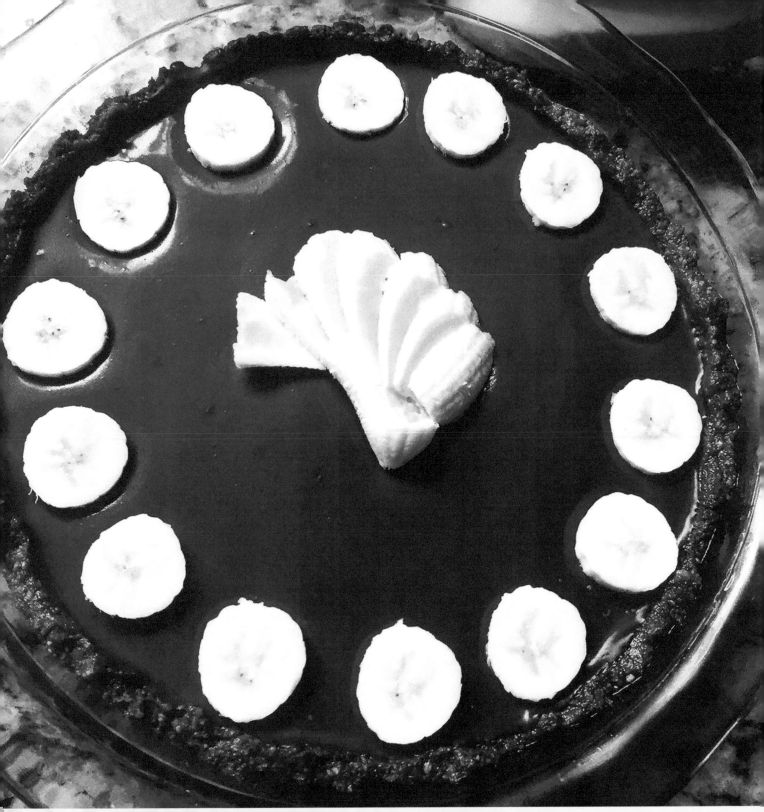

NO CHEESE
RASPBERRY ᵛCHEESECAKE

With simple ingredients and easy prep, you can easily create a gourmet dessert everyone will love. It tastes like raspberry cheesecake but contains no dairy or other processed ingredients, just flavorful whole foods.

TO GET READY:

Round glass pie dish

Blender or food processor

HERE IS WHAT YOU NEED:

Bottom Layer:

1 cup dates

½ cup chopped almonds

1 tablespoon coconut oil

Middle Layer:

2 cups thinly-shredded coconut

1 can coconut cream (paste part only)

1 cup cashews, soaked in water overnight and drained

½ cup water

2 tablespoons maple syrup

1 lemon rind and juice

Top Layer:

2 cups defrosted or fresh raspberries

⅓ cup chia seeds

1 tablespoon maple syrup

LET'S DO THIS:

1. Combine the bottom layer ingredients in a food processor and process until smooth. Spread evenly into the dish, making sure to fill the sides. Place in the freezer for half hour.

2. For the second layer, process the ingredients in a food processor or a high-power blender until very smooth. Pour over the first layer and freeze for 30 minutes.

3. For the top layer, place the raspberries in maple syrup in a sauce pan. Cook on low and mash the raspberries slightly. Take off the stove and add the chia seeds. Let cool and pour over the middle layer. Keep in the refrigerator for a few hours, then move it to the freezer until ready to serve.

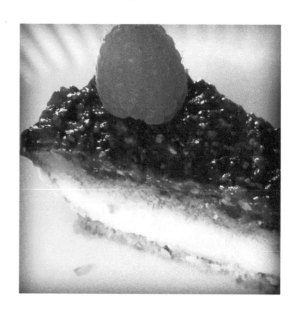

DESSERTS

230

I LIVE IN MY KITCHEN

CHOCOLATE TRUFFLES

Truffles made from "super foods"? Count me in! With just 3 ingredients, this is a super-easy and simple recipe, but it tastes like you spent hours in the kitchen. If you use organic, 85% cocoa dark chocolate, the truffles will also be a very low-sugar treat that is high in antioxidants and healthy fats, which means all taste and no guilt!

TO GET READY:

Rectangular pan lined with parchment paper

Food processor

HERE IS WHAT YOU NEED:

2 packages dark chocolate (8oz.)

1 container raw tahini (16oz.)

Optional: ½ cup chopped walnuts or cocoa powder for garnish

LET'S DO THIS:

1. Pour the raw tahini into a food processor container.

2. Break the chocolate into a saucepan and melt it gently on low heat, being careful not to burn it. Pour the melted chocolate on the tahini and blend well. You may need to stop a few times to scrape the sides of the container, to make sure the mixture is well-combined.

3. Pour the entire mixture onto parchment paper and spread evenly. Refrigerate. Take out and cut into small squares.

Optional: After you spread the mixture into the pan, sprinkle chopped walnuts across the top. Or, sprinkle 1 tablespoon of cocoa powder using a sifter for a nice presentation.

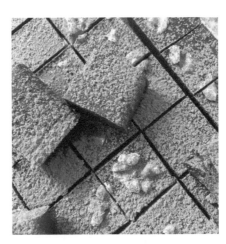

BAKED APPLES

My mom used to make this dish a lot, not just for dessert, but as a snack for us to nosh on and to have around the house. It is a simple and basic recipe with big and delicious results. And most importantly, it is very healthy! I love to make it in the fall when there is an abundance of crispy apples around, but this warming and comforting dish can be made in any season and for any occasion.

TO GET READY:
Oven-safe dish
Heat the oven on 350°F

HERE IS WHAT YOU NEED:
8-10 Granny Smith apples, cored carefully

Filling:
¾ cup coconut sugar
½ cup chopped pecans
½ cup almond meal
1 teaspoon cinnamon
2 tablespoons honey or maple syrup to drizzle on top after baking

LET'S DO THIS:

1. Mix together the filling ingredients in a small bowl and set aside.

2. Cut small slits in the apple skin to prevent them from "exploding" in the oven. Spread out the apples in a baking dish, leaving space between them. Stuff the apple cores with the cinnamon mixture. Use your fingers to push the filling down tightly.

3. Bake at 350°F for 40 minutes. If the apples are relatively small, 30 minutes should be enough. Ideally, the apples will keep their shape and be al dente, not too soft and not too hard.

4. Drizzle all over with 2-3 tablespoons of either honey or maple syrup. You can serve the apples warm or at room temperature. If you really want to get fancy, add a scoop of vanilla ice cream next to the apple.

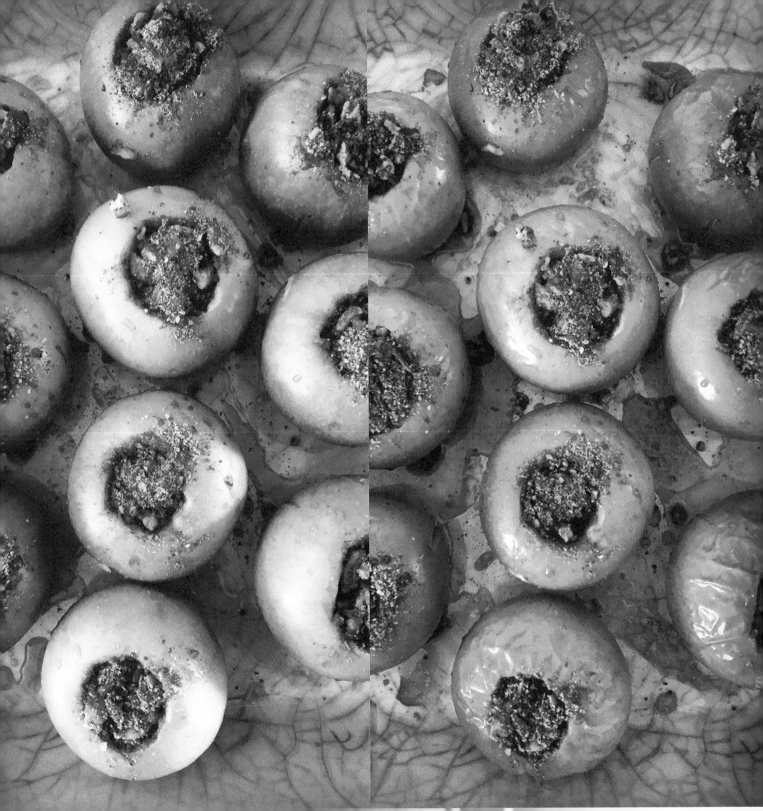

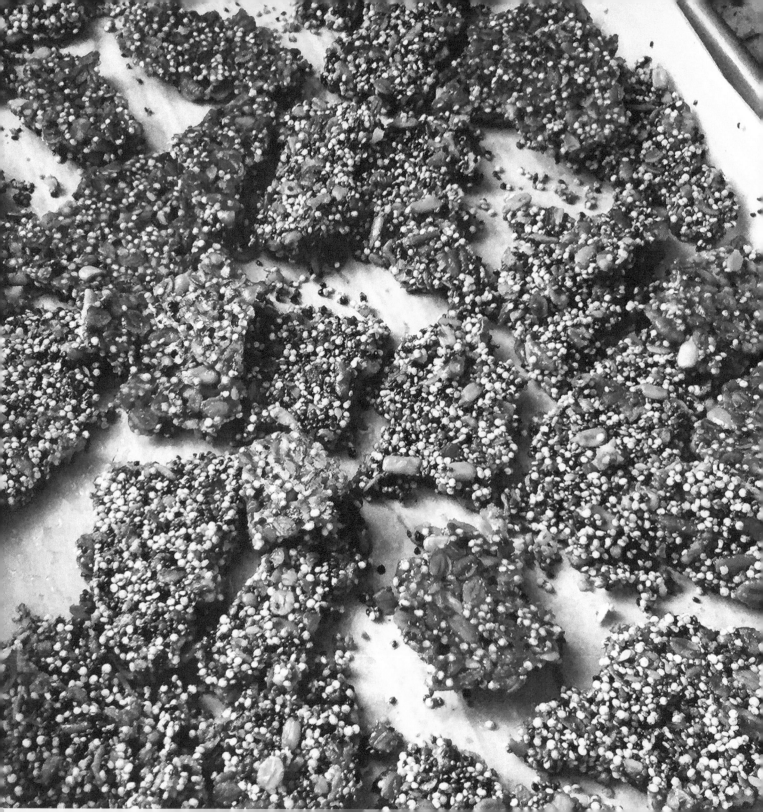

QUINOA BRITTLE

If you are looking for a healthy, crunchy, and sweet treat, you've found it! Keep this brittle around the house for a quick, crunchy and healthy snack, pack it for lunch, or grab it while you are running out the door. They will keep fresh for a couple of weeks in an airtight container on the counter or pantry.

TO GET READY:

Parchment paper

Cookie sheet

Large mixing bowl

Heat the oven to 350°F

HERE IS WHAT YOU NEED:

1 cup dry quinoa (any color)

1 cup pecans, chopped to small pieces

½ cup raw sunflower seeds (can be subbed with oats)

¾ cup oats

¼ teaspoon cinnamon

Sauce:

4 tablespoons coconut oil

½ cup coconut sugar

½ cup maple syrup

Pinch sea salt

LET'S DO THIS:

1. Line a cookie sheet with parchment paper.

2. Combine the quinoa, pecans, sunflower seeds, oats and cinnamon in a large bowl.

3. In a small saucepan on medium-low heat combine the sauce ingredients and stir until it starts bubbling. Take off the stove and pour over the seed mixture. Using a wooden spoon, mix well until everything is coated evenly.

4. Spread the mixture evenly on the parchment paper leaving space to allow the mixture to expand.

5. Bake at 325°F for 15 minutes. Turn the pan and continue baking for another 5 minutes.

6. Let cool for 2 hours. Break into bite size pieces and store in an airtight dish.

NUTS & SEEDS BARS

These bars are great to have around the house as a healthy treat for everyone.

TO GET READY:

Rimmed cookie sheet lined with parchment paper

Heat the oven to 350°F

HERE IS WHAT YOU NEED:

3 cups of raw mixed nuts, such as walnuts, pecans, sunflower seeds, pumpkin seeds, chopped almonds, pistachios and cashews

3 egg whites

1–2 tablespoons maple syrup

Pinch of salt

LET'S DO THIS:

1. Place the nuts in a mixing bowl.

2. In a separate bowl, lightly beat the egg whites with a whisk, add the maple syrup and salt, and pour the mixture over the nuts. Mix everything together very well.

3. Line a cookie sheet with parchment paper. Spread the mix in a thin, flat, even layer and bake at 350°F for 25 minutes. Let it cool completely, then cut with serrated knife or pizza cutter to create small bars. Store them in an airtight container.

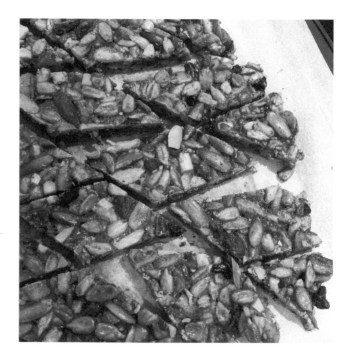

Seeds for Thought...
Did you know that most of the roasted nuts and seeds have added low-grade oil and salt? Buying RAW nuts and seeds is always better option.

AWESOME CHOCOLATE CHIP COOKIES

These cookies are made from wholesome ingredients and they taste just like the cookies from your childhood—or maybe even better!

TO GET READY:

Cookie sheet lined with non-stick baking mat

Mixer

Heat the oven to 350°F

HERE IS WHAT YOU NEED:

¾ cup melted coconut oil or butter (or a combo of both)

¾ cup coconut sugar

2 eggs

1 teaspoon vanilla

1½ cup almond meal

½ cup arrowroot flour

½ cup coconut flour

¼ teaspoon baking soda

Pinch of salt

½ cup chocolate chips (optional: add ¼ cup more)

LET'S DO THIS:

1. In a mixer bowl, blend the oil and sugar at medium speed until a consistent mixture is formed. Reduce the speed and add the eggs, one at a time. Mix for a few minutes, then add the rest of the ingredients until well-combined. Refrigerate for one hour.

2. Using a teaspoon, scoop the dough onto the cookie sheet. Bake at 350°F for 12-14 minutes. Let cool for 15-20 minutes, then transfer to a cooling rack.

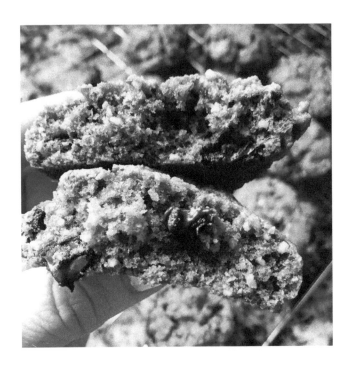

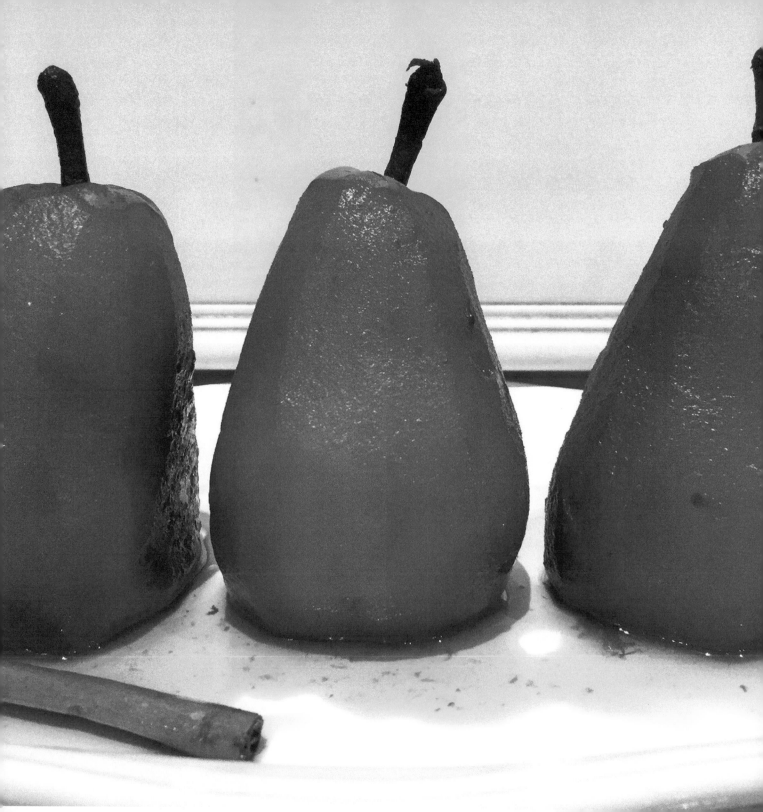

CARAMELIZED PEARS

This recipe is a great ending to a special meal like Thanksgiving dinner. It reminds me of fall and all the flavors that are typical for that season. It uses very simple ingredients yet produces an elegant and delicious dessert. Best of all, you can make it ahead of time and then relax while you are hosting company.

TO GET READY:

Large soup pot

Large glass dish for storage

Serving plate

HERE IS WHAT YOU NEED:

6-8 pears, peeled, with the stems still on

10 prunes

½ cup dried cherries

½ cup dried cranberries

½ cup honey

2 sticks cinnamon

Orange peel (about 1")

LET'S DO THIS:

1. Combine all the ingredients in a pot big enough to submerge the pears in water.

2. Bring the water to a boil. Lower the heat to low and cover. Let simmer for an hour.

3. While cooking, turn the pears every so often, to ensure they have even color. Let the pears cool completely before storing.

4. Serve with a drizzle of the sauce on top of the pears.

239

CHOCOLATE COOKIES

These are light and yummy cookies that you can whip up very quickly and enjoy a chocolate treat without the guilt.

TO GET READY:

Cookie sheet lined with parchment paper or non-stick baking mat

Mixer

Cooling rack

Heat the oven to 350°F

HERE IS WHAT YOU NEED:

4 egg whites

1 cup coconut sugar

Pinch salt

1 tablespoon honey

1 cup almond meal

½ cup cocoa powder

¼ teaspoon baking soda

Optional: Powdered sugar for dusting on top

LET'S DO THIS:

1. In a mixer bowl, beat the egg whites on high speed. When white foam starts to form, gradually add the salt, sugar, and honey. Continue to mix on high speed until the egg whites become firm foam. Set the bowl on the counter.

2. In the meantime, blend the dry ingredients in a separate bowl. Set the two bowls next to each other. Add the dry ingredients slowly to the egg whites in gentle folding motions.

3. Use a spoon to scoop the cookies onto a cookie sheet and bake at 350°F for 12-14 minutes. Let the cookies cool for a few minutes, then transfer them to a cooling rack.

Optional: Sprinkle a thin layer of powdered sugar on the cookies, for a very pretty presentation.

Seeds for Thought... Should you use cocoa or cacao? They are actually two different things. While cacao powder is made using low temps and retains all the health benefits, cocoa powder is made using very high temperatures, which destroys some of its health benefits. However, cocoa powder is less bitter and well-suited for baking and cooking. Both cocoa and cacao contain antioxidants that support your health; just make sure they contain no additional sweeteners or additives.

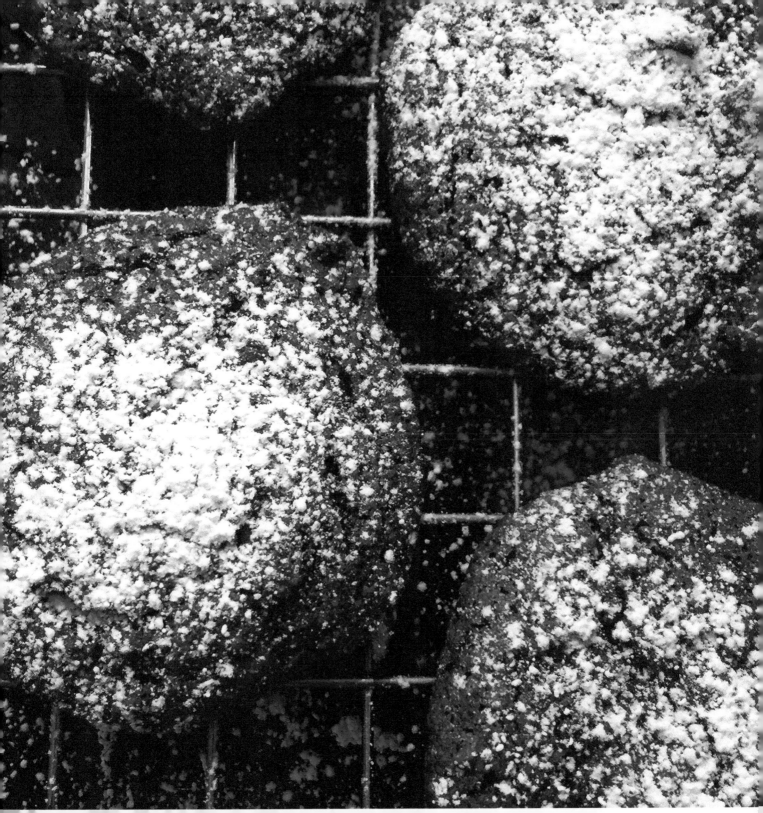

5 MINUTES THUMB COOKIES

This is my go-to recipe when I need a quick dessert that everyone loves. These cookies are perfect to have around the house for when you crave a sweet fix or pack them in a cute box to give as a gift. And best of all, they take 5 minutes to prepare!

TO GET READY:

Rectangular pan lined with parchment paper

Mixer

Heat oven to 350°F

HERE IS WHAT YOU NEED:

¼ cup coconut oil

½ cup coconut sugar

1 egg

1 teaspoon vanilla

2 cups almond flour

Pinch of sea salt

Add a sprinkle of cinnamon or ½ teaspoon of lemon rind (optional)

Filling:

Chocolate chips or strawberry jam

LET'S DO THIS:

1. In a medium bowl mix the oil, sugar, egg and vanilla.

2. Add the almond flour and salt. Optional to add either cinnamon or lemon rind.

3. Mix all together until combined. Form balls with your hands and push with your thumb to create a well. Fill with jam or chocolate chips and bake at 350°F for 8-10 minutes. Let cool on a cooling rack before storing them in a cookie jar.

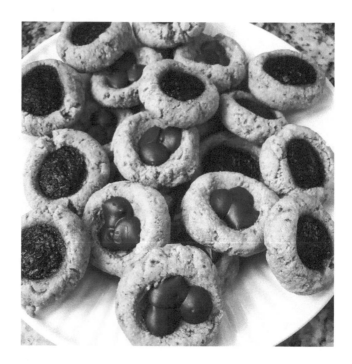

CHOCOLATE MOUSSE

This is a true treat for chocolate lovers but unlike many other recipes, this one uses only wholesome ingredients so you can enjoy it with no guilt at all!

TO GET READY:

Food processor

Small saucepan

4-6 individual glass bowls

HERE IS WHAT YOU NEED:

4 eggs

1 cup coconut milk

1 cup pumpkin paste

½ cup cocoa powder

¼ teaspoon cinnamon

¼ cup coconut sugar

2 cups dark chocolate chips

LET'S DO THIS:

1. Place all the ingredients, except for the chocolate chips, in a food processor.

2. Melt the chocolate chips in a small saucepan on very low heat, mixing it consistently until a smooth chocolate sauce forms. Pour the chocolate over the ingredients in the food processor and blend for a couple of minutes.

3. Divide the mixture between 4 or 6 small glass dishes and refrigerate for at least 1-2 hours. Alternately, you can pour everything to one glass dish and scoop to individual portions later on.

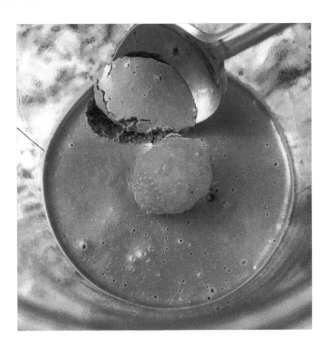

CHOCOLATE CHIP BANANA MUFFINS

These little treats are delicious and very simple to make. In fact, it is so easy that you won't even have to use the mixer, just a mixing bowl and a spoon. It is a great recipe to get the kids involved; they can start by mashing the bananas with a fork, fill up a cup with chocolate chips, or simply lick the bowl. Let them discover the fun in baking!

TO GET READY:

Large mixing bowl

Muffin pan with liners

Whisk or potato masher

Heat the oven to 350°F

HERE IS WHAT YOU NEED:

2 bananas, mashed with a fork

3 eggs

¼ cup coconut sugar

⅓ cup kefir or Greek yogurt

½ cup spelt flour

1 cup almond flour

¼ teaspoon baking soda

¼ teaspoon baking powder

Pinch salt

¾-1 cup chocolate chips

LET'S DO THIS:

1. In a large mixing bowl mash the bananas with a fork. Add the eggs and mix well. Add the rest of the ingredients, except for the chocolate chips, stir to incorporate everything to a smooth batter. Lastly, add the chocolate chips and blend them in.

2. Line muffin pan with 12 paper liners and bake at 350°F for 25 minutes, or use a mini muffin pan with 24 paper liners and bake at 350°F for 20 minutes.

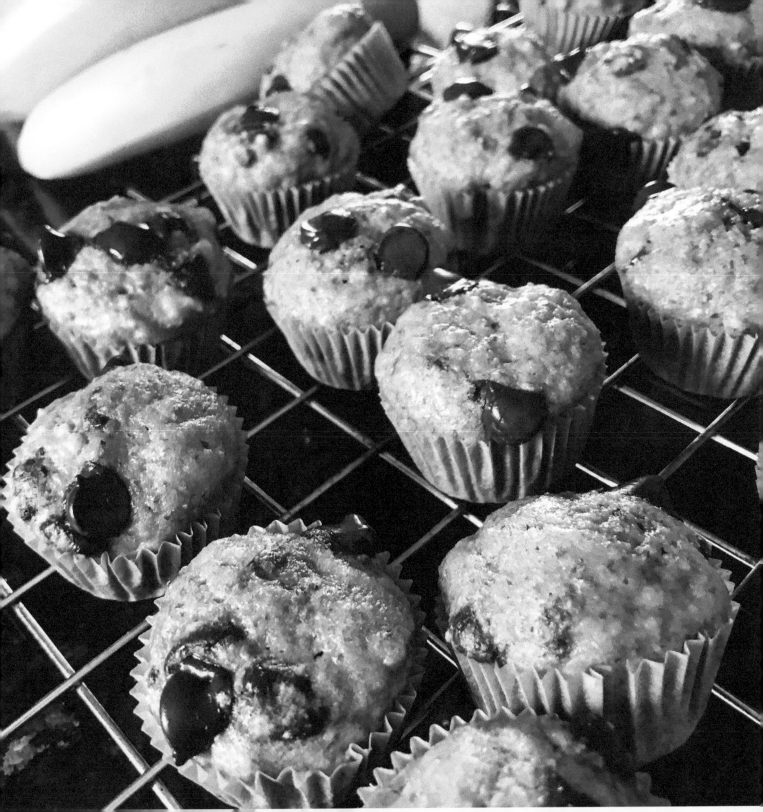

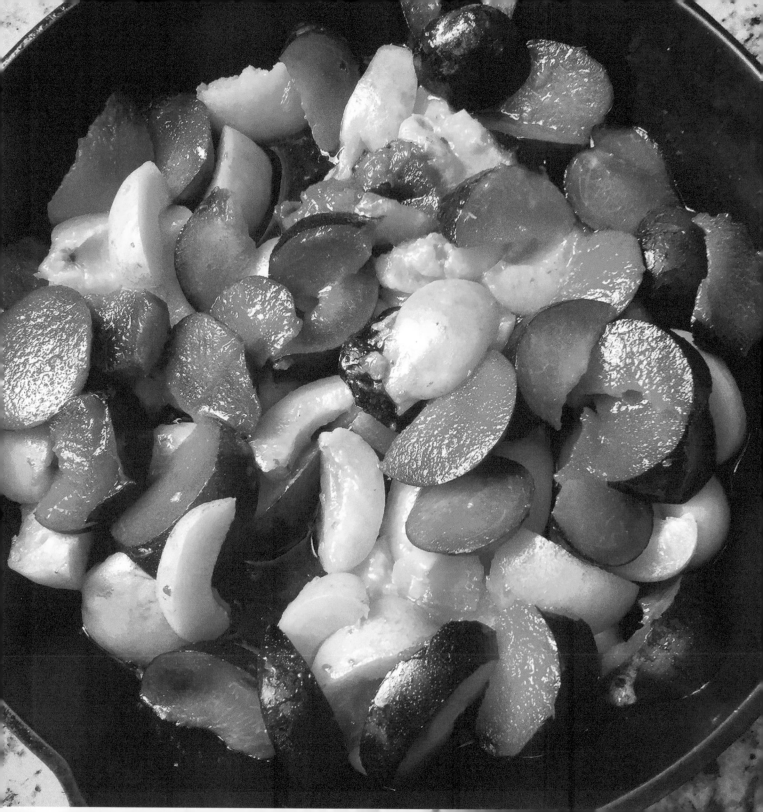

PLUMS'N PEACHES COBBLER

This is a great dessert for the summer, when plums and peaches are in season and can be found at any farmer's market. It has beautiful colors and the flavors are absolutely divine. You can serve this cobbler while it is still warm with a scoop of (healthy) ice cream, but it is absolutely heavenly by itself.

TO GET READY:

Cast-iron skillet or any skillet

Round ceramic dish (if not using a cast-iron skillet)

Medium mixing bowl

Heat the oven to 350°F

HERE IS WHAT YOU NEED:

6 peaches, cut into wedges

6 plums, cut into wedges

1 tablespoon coconut oil

Batter:

3 eggs

¼ cup olive oil

⅓ cup coconut sugar

1 cup almond flour

2 tablespoons arrowroot flour

¼ teaspoon baking soda

¼ teaspoon baking powder

½ teaspoon cinnamon

1 tablespoon vanilla

2 tablespoons coconut sugar to use as a garnish, before baking

LET'S DO THIS:

1. Heat the oil in a skillet on medium-low and add the fruit. Cook for 5 minutes until just a little bubbly. Turn off the heat. Make sure not to overcook, as this will cause the fruit to be too soft.

2. While the fruit is cooking, add the rest of the ingredients to a bowl and mix well to create the batter.

3. Pour the fruit into a round, greased baking dish, and pour the batter over the fruit. Swirl the two together just until you have a marbled pattern. Sprinkle the coconut sugar on top.

4. Bake on 350°F for 30 minutes.

Optional: If you have a cast-iron skillet, try this variation. After the fruits are cooked a bit and the batter is ready in a separate bowl, pour the batter on top of the fruits. Swirl the two together just until you have a marbled pattern. Cook on the stove for 10 more minutes on low heat, then transfer to a 350°F oven for 20 more minutes.

IT'S BETTER THAN ICE CREAM— IT'S NICE CREAM!

Who doesn't like ice cream? But we were told that ice cream was bad for us, especially if we were trying to improve our health. There are many brands of ice cream available, but each contains at least one or two unhealthy ingredients like white sugar, soy or any other artificial ingredient that makes it creamier, sweeter, with a longer shelf life. The following recipes are easy enough to make Nice Cream at home in just a few minutes with only a few basic ingredients; no ice cream maker is necessary. The recipes all use a high-power blender, which is a great investment for any kitchen. Use your imagination and custom-build your Nice Cream to suit your taste buds. As always, have fun with it!

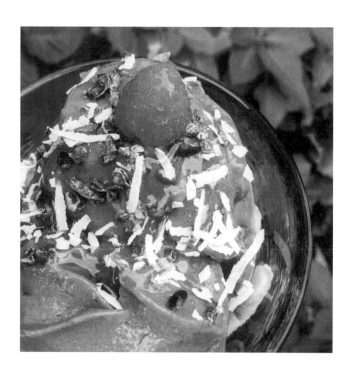

Seeds for Thought...
Never throw away "old" fruits.
Simply clean, peel, pit, cut, and place
in a Ziploc® bag in the freezer for a
future smoothie or Nice Cream.

CHOCOLATE NICE CREAM

Yes, please! This recipe is for all you chocolate lovers, a frozen treat with no added chemicals or refined sugars. In fact, it is actually good for you! So, what are you waiting for?

TO GET READY:

High-power blender
  or food processor

HERE IS WHAT YOU NEED:

1 frozen banana

1 frozen avocado (pitted
  and peeled, frozen ahead
  of time)

¼ cup water (or nut milk)

¼ cup almond meal

⅓ cup coconut sugar

¼ cup cocoa powder

Pecans or walnuts,
  for garnish (optional)

LET'S DO THIS:

1. Combine all of the ingredients in a food processor on low speed for a few seconds. Turn the machine to high speed and process until smooth. You might have to stop a couple of times and scrape the mixture from the walls of the blender and process again.

2. Transfer to a glass dish and freeze for an hour or two before serving.

Optional: garnish with pecans or walnuts, for a little crunch.

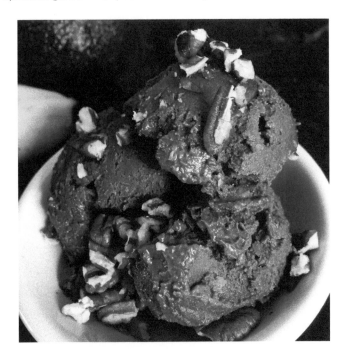

COFFEE NICE CREAM

If you love the taste of coffee as much as I do, now you can enjoy it as a delicous and nutritious ice cream. In fact, it can be your next healthy breakfast!

TO GET READY:

High-power blender
   or food processor

HERE IS WHAT YOU NEED:

1 cup freshly-brewed
   coffee, frozen

½ cup cashews (soaked in
   water overnight and drained)

1 tablespoon coconut oil

½ cup cooked white quinoa

2 frozen bananas

LET'S DO THIS:

Blend all the ingredients in a high power blender and serve immediately or freeze for later use.

Optional: Can be garnished with cocoa nibs, melted chocolate, maple syrup, honey, cinnamon, etc. Mmmm, mmmmm, mmmmmm...

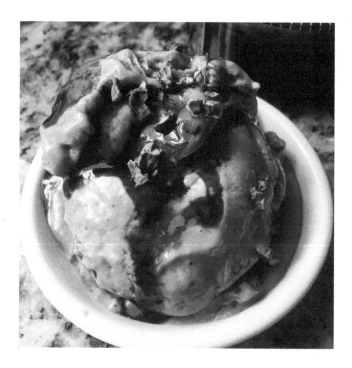

BLUEBERRY NICE CREAM

With just four ingredients, you can make homemade ice cream that tastes as good as a blueberry pie!

TO GET READY:

High-power blender
or food processor

HERE IS WHAT YOU NEED:

2 cups organic Kefir

2 cups organic frozen
  blueberries

2 tablespoons organic
  maple syrup

1 frozen banana

2 handfuls walnuts

or

½ cup almond butter

or

½ cup cashew butter

LET'S DO THIS:

1. Combine all the ingredients in a food processor bowl and process until smooth.

2. Store in a glass container for about 2 hours in the freezer. Keep frozen and take out half hour before serving so it softens a little. If you like your ice cream sweeter, add more maple syrup or honey.

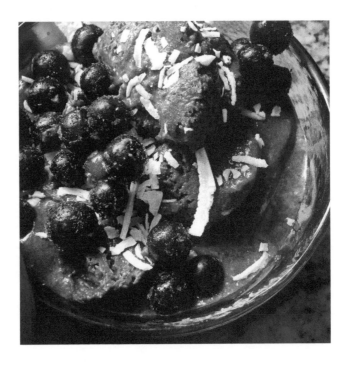

RASPBERRY NICE CREAM

This Nice Cream is not only beautiful, but it is made from wholesome and nourishing ingredients only.

TO GET READY:

High-power blender
  or food processor

HERE IS WHAT YOU NEED:

1 banana (preferred frozen)

1 frozen avocado

1 bag frozen raspberries (12oz.)

1 tablespoon coconut oil

2 tablespoons maple syrup

LET'S DO THIS:

Combine all ingredients together in a high power blender.

Serve immediately or store in a glass container in the freezer. Defrost for a half hour before serving.

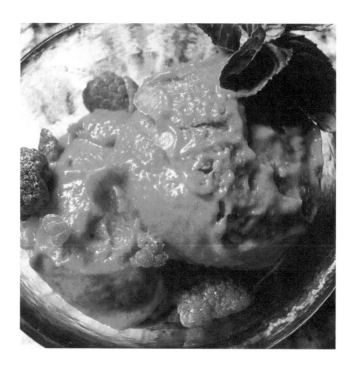

MANGO NICE CREAM

With just 3 ingredients, create an ice cream that will keep you both happy and healthy.

TO GET READY:

High-power blender
  or food processor

HERE IS WHAT YOU NEED:

2 cups frozen mango chunks

2 cups frozen peaches

1 can coconut milk (refrigerated)

LET'S DO THIS:

1. Use a high-power blender to blend all of the ingredients.

2. Enjoy immediately, or store in the freezer for later use in a glass dish. Be sure to take it out of the freezer about half hour before serving, so it is soft enough to scoop.

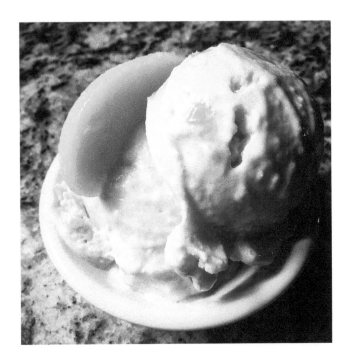

THANK YOU

Thank you to my husband and best friend, Arik,
who always supports and encourages me to do what I love.

To my children, Eden, Adee, and Amit, for being my biggest fans
and inspiration for my work.

To my sister, Sagit, who encouraged me to document my cooking,
Thank you.

I love you all so very much!

CPSIA information can be obtained
at www.ICGtesting.com
Printed in the USA
LVHW07n1245041018
592382LV00006B/22/P

9 780692 869796